mike
with very best wishes

Bill

—A Handbook of—
HYPERLIPIDAEMIA

by GR Thompson (London)

Advisory Board
L Carlson (Stockholm)
DR Illingworth (Portland)
E Stein (Cincinnati)
G Utermann (Innsbruck)

MSD
MERCK
SHARP &
DOHME

Produced and published by CURRENT SCIENCE

Published by Current Science Ltd, London

12-90 MVC 88-R-3159B-CCS

British Library Cataloguing-in-Publication Data:

Thompson, G.R.
    A handbook of hyperlipidaemia.
    1. Man. Blood. Hyperlipidaemia
    I. Title
    616.3997

ISBN 1-870485-16-5

Printed in Spain by Imago Publishing Ltd

FOREWORD

Lipoprotein traffic — navigating the maze

Like the London Underground, the lipoprotein transport system shuttles its passenger lipids; cholesterol and triglycerides, from place to place. Rush hour occurs after eating, when lipids flood the bloodstream from the intestine. Like passengers on the Underground, the lipids exchange from one carrier to another before reaching their final destinations. At times these exchanges produce transient overloading of particular carriers. Frequently, a lipid is delivered to one organ, only to emerge somewhat later for delivery to a new organ. This incessant recycling keeps traffic moving even when food is not ingested.

Traffic jams develop in the lipoprotein transport system as they do on the Underground. Some of these blocks are determined genetically, like design flaws in the Underground. More commonly, a blockage occurs when a pathway of marginal capacity is overloaded with excess traffic. This situation pertains in multifactorial hyperlipidaemia when dietary or endocrine imbalances overwhelm the lipid transport system and produce hyperlipidaemia in genetically susceptible people.

Traffic blocks in the lipoprotein transport system can now be detected and opened up or bypassed. The input of passenger lipids can be diminished by a low-fat diet, or by nicotinic acid, which blocks the recycling of fatty acids from adipose tissue to liver. Traffic flow can be accelerated by drugs such as bile acid binding resins and HMG CoA reductase inhibitors, which enhance the receptor-dependent removal of lipoproteins from blood. Even when the level of lipoproteins cannot be reduced sufficiently, it may be possible to prevent arterial damage by preventing lipid oxidation and protein modification. In view of this progress, it seems likely that most of the medical problems in lipid transport will be solved long before the traffic problems in the London Underground are abolished.

Just as a traveller would have difficulty negotiating the London Underground without a map, the physician will have difficulty in circumventing lipid road blocks unless he understands the routes of traffic. Progress in this field has been so rapid that most physicians have not yet absorbed the advances or put them into practical use. This handbook will help to solve that problem. Like a guide to the Underground, this handbook should allow the informed physician to manoeuvre through the complex maze of lipoprotein and lipid traffic. Clearly written, the book delineates the normal routes of lipid transport, signals the roadblocks, and proposes a rational approach to prevention and therapy. As the contents of this book become widely disseminated, clinical awareness of problems in lipid transport will broaden, and physicians will gain the confidence needed to navigate this maze with ease.

Michael S. Brown
Joseph L. Goldstein
Dallas, Texas

CONTENTS

Abbreviations used in this book

ACAT	acyl: cholesterol acyltransferase
ACE	angiotensin converting enzyme
AHA	American Heart Association
apoA	apolipoprotein A
apoB	apolipoprotein B
apoC	apolipoprotein C
apoD	apolipoprotein D
apoE	apolipoprotein E
BCS	British Cardiac Society
BHA	British Heart Association
BUPA	British United Provident Association
CABG	coronary artery bypass graft
CAPD	chronic ambulatory peritoneal dialysis
CDC	Centers for Disease Control
CE	cholesterol ester
CETP	cholesterol ester transferase protein
CHD	coronary heart disease
CLAS	Cholesterol Lowering Atherosclerosis Study
COMA	Committee on the Medical Aspects of Food Policy
CPK	creatine phosphokinase
d	density
DHA	docosahexaenoic acid
EAS	European Atherosclerosis Society
ECG	electrocardiogram
EIA	electroimmunoassay
ELISA	enzyme-linked immunosorbent assay
EPA	eicosapentaenoic acid
FC	free cholesterol
FCH	familial combined hyperlipidaemia
FFA	free fatty acid
FFP	fresh frozen plasma
FH	familial hypercholesterolaemia
γGT	gamma-glutamyl transpeptidase
HbA_1	haemoglobin A_1
HDL	high-density lipoprotein
HDLC	high-density lipoprotein cholesterol
HELP	Heparin Extracorporeal LDL Precipitation [system]
HMG CoA	β-hydroxy-β-methylglutaryl-coenzyme A
HPL	hepatic lipase
hyperapoB	hyperapoβlipoproteinaemia
IDDM	insulin-dependent diabetes mellitus
IDL	intermediate-density lipoprotein
IHD	ischaemic heart disease
ISA	intrinsic sympathomimetic activity
LCAT	lecithin: cholesterol acyltransferase

LDL	low-density lipoprotein
LRC	Lipid Research Clinics
LSI	light scattering index
MI	myocardial infarction
MRFIT	Multiple Risk Factor Intervention Trial
NCEP	National Cholesterol Education Program
NHLBI	National Heart Lung and Blood Institute
NIH	National Institutes of Health
PDGF	platelet-derived growth factor
PHLA	post-heparin lipolytic activity
PIB	partial ileal bypass
PL	phospholipid
PPF	plasma protein fraction
P : S	the ratio of polyunsaturated to saturated fatty acids
RFLP	restriction fragment length polymorphism
RID	radial immunodiffusion
S_f	flotation rate
TC	total cholesterol
TG	triglyceride
TMU	tetramethylurea
TSH	thyroid-stimulating hormone
VLDL	very-low-density lipoprotein
WHHL	Watanabe heritable hyperlipidaemia [rabbit]
WHO	World Health Organization

Conversion of cholesterol and triglyceride values

From mg/dl to mmol/l:
    for cholesterol divide mg/dl by 38.7
    for triglyceride divide mg/dl by 88.5
From mmol/l to mg/dl:
    for cholesterol multiply mmol/l by 38.7
    for triglyceride multiply mmol/l by 88.5

INTRODUCTION

This handbook is intended both for those who know nothing about lipids and for those who know something but would like to learn more. It is too large to be a pocket handbook but not large enough to qualify as a work of reference. However, readers requiring more detail can always refer to what I consider to be the key papers published on lipids since I first took an interest in the subject 25 years ago. This interest started here at the Hammersmith Hospital, London, and was encouraged there initially by Barry Lewis and Nick Myant. It burgeoned in Boston in 1966–1967 while I was a research fellow with Kurt Isselbacher and matured further during a year's leave of absence in Houston with Tony Gotto. The book reflects many of the ideas and attitudes that I acquired from these and other colleagues who influenced me during a journey which started in the gastrointestinal tract and ended up in the arterial wall. I am grateful to all of them for helping me, in the words of Robert Frost, to take the road 'less travelled by, and that has made all the difference'.

More immediately I am grateful to Mike Brown and Joe Goldstein for their witty and perceptive foreword, and to the four members of my Advisory Board, who devoted considerable time and effort to improving the book. Gerd Utermann reviewed Chapters 1 and 5; Lars Carlson, Chapters 2, 7, 9 and 14; Evan Stein, Chapters 3, 4 and 6; and Roger Illingworth, Chapters 8, 10, 11 and 12. I am grateful also to my publishers, Current Science, especially Anne Greenwood and Caroline Black, who persuaded and helped me to write this book, and last but certainly not least, to my secretary Elizabeth Manson who translated my pencilled scrawl into aptly named 'Word Perfect' typescript with commendable speed, precision and willingness.

Gilbert Thompson
Hammersmith Hospital
London

Plasma lipids

Introduction

The major lipids found in human plasma are triglycerides, phospholipids and cholesterol esters. These molecules are all esters of long-chain fatty acids, and together they comprise the lipid moiety of lipoproteins. Fatty acids also exist in plasma in the free (non-esterified) form. The major fatty acids found in plasma in either the free or esterified form are listed in Table 1.1.

Linoleic acid cannot be synthesized by animals and hence is an essential fatty acid, as is its metabolic product, arachidonic acid. Most of the remaining fatty acids can be synthesized by the liver from carbohydrate precursors, a process involving elongation and, in some instances, desaturation of fatty acyl chains by microsomal enzymes.

Free fatty acids

Free fatty acids (FFA) are the form in which fatty acids are transported from their storage site in adipose tissue to their sites of utilization in the liver and

1

Table 1.1. Fatty acids found in human plasma.

Common name	Abbreviated formula
Myristic acid	C14:0
Palmitic acid	C16:0
Palmitoleic acid	C16:1ω7
Stearic acid	C18:0
Oleic acid	C18:1ω9
Linoleic acid	C18:2ω6
Arachidonic acid	C20:4ω6
Eicosapentaenoic acid	C20:5ω3
Docosahexaenoic acid	C22:6ω3

The abbreviated formula gives the number of carbon atoms and the number of double bonds. The location of the double bond nearest to the methyl terminus, counting from same, is indicated by the symbol ω.

muscle. Fatty acids are stored in adipose tissue as triglycerides, especially palmitic, oleic and linoleic acids. The rate-limiting step in the mobilization of this triglyceride is a hormone-sensitive lipase, the activity of which is enhanced by hormones such as noradrenaline and the glucocorticoids. Lipolysis results in release of FFA and glycerol into plasma and is promoted by acute stress, prolonged fasting and insulin lack.

The concentration of FFA in human plasma normally ranges from 0.4 to 0.8 mmol/l, most of which is bound to albumin. The fractional rate of turnover of FFA is extremely rapid, 20–40% of the total mass entering plasma being utilized every minute to undergo oxidation, re-esterification or conversion to other fatty acids. Major sites of oxidation are the liver and heart, in the resting state, and skeletal muscle during exercise, when the proportion oxidized rises from about 20 to 60%. Much of the FFA taken up by the liver undergoes re-esterification, chiefly to triglyceride but also to phospholipid, especially in the case of linoleic acid.

Triglycerides

Triglycerides, or triacylglycerols, are fatty acid esters of glycerol, usually containing a mixture of two or three different fatty acids. Stereospecific analysis shows that palmitic acid preferentially occupies the 1-position in the molecule, linoleic acid the 2-position, and oleic acid the 3-position. Synthesis of triglycerides in the liver and in adipose tissue occurs via the glycerol phosphate pathway [1] whereas synthesis in the small intestine during fat absorption proceeds mainly via the monoglyceride pathway [2].

Dietary triglycerides are absorbed mainly in the form of chylomicrons which traverse the intestinal lymphatics and enter the systemic circulation via the

1

thoracic duct. Normally, over 90% of triglyceride is absorbed, which means that roughly 80–170 mmol (70–150 g) of exogenous triglyceride enters the circulation per day. Triglycerides derived from endogenous fatty acid also originate in the small intestine but their chief source is the liver, whence they are secreted in the form of very-low-density lipoproteins (VLDL). The fatty acid pattern of triglycerides in both chylomicrons and VLDL is markedly influenced by the fatty acid composition of dietary triglyceride. If the linoleic acid content of the diet is inadequate, essential fatty acid deficiency can occur, especially in patients with malabsorption [3].

Triglycerides have a relatively short half-life in plasma and are removed by a process involving hydrolysis and uptake by various organs, notably adipose tissue. These events are mediated by lipolytic enzymes, as discussed in Chapter 2. Triglyceride levels remain elevated for several hours after ingestion of a fatty meal but normally all chylomicron triglyceride should have been cleared within 12 hours. Thus, measurement of plasma levels in the fasting state reflects the amount of endogenous triglyceride in the circulation. Normal values for adult males range from 0.5 to 2 mmol/l and up to 1.5 mmol/l in premenopausal females.

Phospholipids
The two main phospholipids found in plasma are phosphatidylcholine (lecithin) and sphingomyelin. Phospholipid synthesis takes place in most tissues, but plasma phospholipids are derived mainly from the liver. The small intestine makes a contribution in the form of chylomicron lecithin. Most of the phospholipid entering the small intestine in the diet or as bile undergoes hydrolysis by pancreatic lipase, which explains why oral supplements of polyunsaturated lecithin do not exert any greater effect on the linoleate content of plasma phospholipids than an equivalent dose of triglyceride in the form of corn oil.

Phospholipids are integral components of all cell membranes and considerable exchange of phosphatidyl choline and sphingomyelin takes place between plasma and red cells. Both these phospholipids exist in plasma as constituents of lipoproteins, where they play a key role in maintaining nonpolar lipids, such as triglycerides and cholesterol esters, in a soluble state. This property reflects the amphipathic nature of phospholipid molecules, their non-polar fatty acyl chains being able to interact with a lipid environment whereas their polar head groups can interact with an aqueous environment [4].

As with plasma triglycerides the fatty acid composition of phospholipids is markedly influenced by the nature of the fat in the diet. Changes in the fatty acid composition of lecithin lead to analogous changes in cholesterol ester composition and this may have some bearing on the mechanism whereby dietary fats influence serum cholesterol levels.

1

Serum phospholipid levels range from 2.3 to 3.0 mmol/l in healthy subjects, being somewhat higher in females than in males. Marked elevations occur in patients with biliary obstruction.

Cholesterol

Cholesterol is a sterol, possessing a four-ringed steroid nucleus and a hydroxyl group. It occurs in man both as the free sterol and esterified with one of several long-chain fatty acids. Free cholesterol is a component of all cell membranes and is the principal form in which cholesterol is present in most tissues. Exceptions are the adrenal cortex, the plasma and atheromatous plaques, where cholesterol esters predominate. In addition, a significant proportion of the cholesterol in intestinal lymph and in the liver is esterified. Most tissues have the capacity to synthesize cholesterol but, under normal circumstances, virtually all the newly synthesized cholesterol in the body originates from the liver and distal part of the small intestine.

An early stage of cholesterol synthesis is the conversion of acetate to mevalonic acid. The rate-limiting enzyme regulating this step is β-hydroxy-β-methylglutaryl-coenzyme A reductase (HMG CoA reductase), which is subject to feedback suppression by its final end-product, cholesterol. The major metabolites of cholesterol are the bile acids, which are synthesized exclusively by the liver, the rate-limiting enzyme here being cholesterol-7-α-hydroxylase.

Long-term studies of changes in plasma-specific activity after the injection of radioactive cholesterol suggest the existence of three body pools of cholesterol, all in equilibrium with plasma cholesterol but with widely differing rates of equilibration (Fig. 1.1). The rapidly exchangeable pool probably represents the cholesterol in plasma lipoproteins, erythrocytes, liver, intestines and certain other viscera, and contains 50–65 mmol (20–25 g). The intermediate pool contains about 25 mmol (10–12 g) and probably represents cholesterol in peripheral tissues such as skin and adipose tissue. The slowly exchangeable pool is the largest, at 90 mmol (35–36 g), and represents cholesterol in a variety of tissues including skeletal muscle and the arterial wall. In addition, there is a non-exchangeable pool in the central nervous system, comprising 35–40% of total body cholesterol [5].

In the metabolic steady state, all input of cholesterol into the rapidly exchangeable pool, that is synthesis plus absorption, will be balanced by outflow, namely faecal excretion. Normally, the latter is approximately 2.9 mmol (1.1 g) per day, 60% of which is in the form of neutral sterols, the remainder as bile acids. The absorption of cholesterol averages 35–40% over a fairly wide range of intake and is mediated via the lymphatic pathway. Absorption of dietary cholesterol and reabsorption of biliary cholesterol play an important role in limiting the rate of hepatic cholesterol synthesis [6]. Bile acid synthesis is regulated by the enterohepatic circulation of bile acids and is de-repressed by any manoeuvre that interferes with their reabsorption.

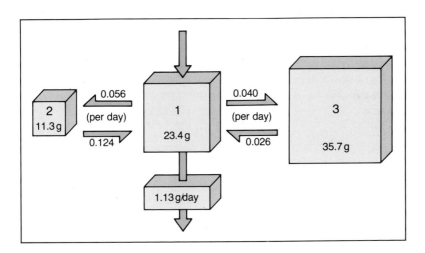

Fig. 1.1. Three-pool model of cholesterol turnover in man. The rate constants of transfer between the rapidly exchangeable (1), intermediate (2) and slowly exchangeable pools (3) are shown, together with the mass of cholesterol in each pool, assuming that all newly synthesized cholesterol enters the rapidly exchangeable pool. Adapted by permission from Goodman *et al., J Lipid Res* 1973, 14:178–188.

More than two-thirds of the cholesterol in plasma is esterified, the predominant esters being cholesterol linoleate and cholesterol oleate. These are formed in plasma by the action of the enzyme lecithin : cholesterol acyltransferase (LCAT) with minor contributions from the enzyme acyl : cholesterol acyltransferase (ACAT) in the small intestine and the liver. The nature of the cholesterol esters is largely determined by the fatty acid composition of plasma lecithin and thus by the type of fat in the diet. In contrast to cholesterol esters, plasma free cholesterol readily exchanges with cholesterol in cell membranes.

Plasma total cholesterol normally ranges between 4 and 6.5 mmol/l but, unlike triglycerides, cholesterol levels do not rise acutely after a fatty meal.

Plasma lipoproteins

Transport
All lipids, except FFA, are transported in plasma in the form of lipoproteins. These macromolecular complexes contain specific apolipoproteins, or

1

apoproteins, which interact with phospholipids and free cholesterol to form the polar, outer shell of lipoprotein particles, encompassing a non-polar core containing triglycerides and cholesterol esters.

By means of preparative ultracentrifugation six distinct classes of lipoprotein can be isolated from postprandial plasma. These are spherical particles which vary in size (Fig. 1.2) and contain a mixture of protein, phospholipid, free and esterified cholesterol and triglyceride, but in markedly different proportions (Table 1.2). They also differ in other respects and these features together with details of their metabolism will be dealt with in Chapter 2. At this stage we will limit ourselves to discussing the distribution of plasma lipids within each of the lipoprotein classes.

As shown in Fig. 1.3, most of the cholesterol in the plasma of fasting normal subjects is carried by low-density lipoprotein (LDL), much smaller proportions being found in VLDL and high-density lipoprotein (HDL). In contrast, most of the endogenous triglyceride is carried by VLDL. Chylomicrons transport dietary triglyceride for a few hours after each meal but are virtually absent from normal plasma after a 12-hour fast. Thus measurement of the total cholesterol and triglyceride content of plasma or serum gives the sum of the contributions from each lipoprotein class. Changes in serum lipids usually reflect changes in lipoprotein concentration but changes in lipoprotein composition can also exert an influence in this respect. Under normal circumstances the concentration of intermediate-density lipoprotein (IDL) or remnant particles in plasma is relatively low, and is usually ignored, but this can become a major determinant of both serum cholesterol and triglyceride in certain forms of hyperlipidaemia.

Physiological influences

Plasma lipid and lipoprotein levels are markedly influenced by intrinsic characteristics such as age, gender and inherited traits, as well as by modifiable factors such as diet, body weight and physical activity. Often it is difficult to discriminate between them since, for example, ageing is frequently accompanied by an increase in body weight and a decrease in physical activity. Nevertheless we will now examine each of these influences in turn and attempt to assess their relative contribution to the variability in serum lipids which occurs both within and between different populations.

Age

Plasma lipid concentrations and lipoprotein distribution at birth differ considerably from the patterns seen in later life. Total cholesterol levels in cord blood averaged 1.65 mmol/l in two American studies, equally distributed between LDL and HDL but with relatively little in VLDL, as reflected by a mean triglyceride of only 0.41 mmol/l. The 95th percentile for LDL cholesterol in cord blood in these studies was 1.05 mmol/l. A rapid rise in serum cholesterol occurs during the first 6 months of life but thereafter there is little change until puberty, cholesterol and triglyceride levels averaging 4 and 0.65 mmol/l,

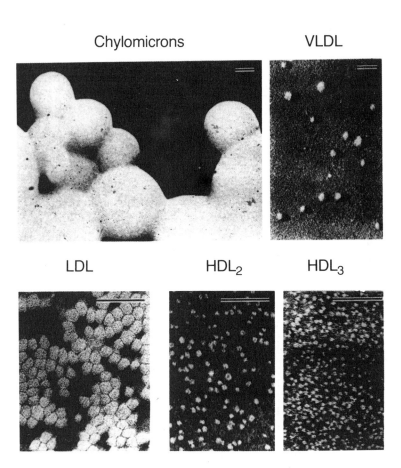

Fig. 1.2. Electron micrographs of the major classes of lipoprotein found in human plasma. Chylomicrons and VLDL were fixed in osmium tetroxide and shadowed with platinum-palladium-gold alloy. LDL and HDL were negatively stained with sodium phospho-tungstate. HDL is subdivided into HDL_2 and the smaller HDL_3 particles. Note the change in scale of the marker which represents 0.1 μm in all instances. Published by permission from Nichols, *Proc Natl Acad Sci USA* 1969, 64:1128–1137.

respectively, over this period. After the age of 15 there is a rise in triglyceride and LDL cholesterol in both sexes and a fall in HDL cholesterol in boys but not in girls [8].

During adult life plasma lipid levels continue to rise in both sexes, the concentration of cholesterol being higher in men up to the age of 55, but higher

Table 1.2. Lipid composition of plasma lipoproteins (after Thompson [7]).

	Chylo-microns	VLDL	IDL*	LDL	HDL$_2$	HDL$_3$
% of total lipoprotein						
Protein	1–2	10	18	25	40	55
Lipid	98–99	90	82	75	60	45
% of total lipids						
Triglyceride	88	56	32	7	6	7
Cholesterol	3	17	41	59	43	38
Phospholipid	9	19	27	28	42	41
% of cholesterol esterified	46	57	66	70	74	81

*Data from Lee and Alaupovic, *Biochemistry* 1970, 9:2244–2252.

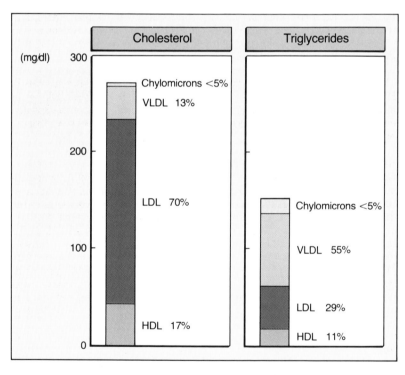

Fig. 1.3. Contribution of each major lipoprotein class to plasma total cholesterol and triglyceride in the normal subject. To convert the scale into mmol/l, divide mg/dl by 38.7 for cholesterol or 88.5 for triglyceride. Adapted by permission from Lees and Wilson, *N Engl J Med* 1971, 284:186–195.

in women thereafter. Triglycerides remain higher in men until the age of 65 when they become similar in both sexes [9]. The rise in total cholesterol mainly reflects an increase in LDL cholesterol, whereas HDL cholesterol levels remain relatively constant in males (Fig. 1.4). In women HDL cholesterol levels are higher than in men at all ages from puberty onwards and do not decrease after the menopause. Studies within families show that rises in total cholesterol, triglyceride and LDL cholesterol remain correlated with age even after correcting for the increases in body weight which occur [10]. There is evidence that the rise in LDL cholesterol with age reflects a progressive decrease in LDL catabolism which, particularly in women, could reflect hormonal changes.

Gender

Some of the male–female differences have already been touched upon. Females tend to have lower triglyceride and VLDL cholesterol levels and higher HDL cholesterol levels than men from puberty onwards. Their total and LDL cholesterol levels are lower until the menopause but thereafter become higher than in men of similar age (Fig. 1.4), except for women taking hormone replacement therapy. Females of all ages who are on oestrogens and/or progestogens tend to have higher triglycerides but lower levels of LDL than those not on hormones [9].

The higher HDL cholesterol of females reflects a higher concentration of HDL_2 in plasma, HDL_3 concentrations being similar in both sexes. Differences in endogenous sex hormones presumably account for much of these differences, oestrogens tending to lower LDL and raise HDL whereas androgens have the opposite effect.

Race

Here again it is difficult to separate genetically determined from environmental influences such as diet and physical activity. For example, the Japanese have higher HDL cholesterol levels than those found in Western countries but this difference is no longer evident if the comparison is made with Westerners living in Japan, presumably because they are eating a Japanese diet. The Lipid Research Clinics (LRC) Prevalence Study showed that black American males have a higher HDL : total cholesterol ratio than their white counterparts [11] and a similar tendency has been reported in international comparisons between African and European countries. This may therefore represent a genuine racial trait in those of African origin although it should be noted that in black females in the LRC Prevalence Study a higher HDL : total cholesterol ratio was seen only below the age of 20.

Body weight

Several studies have shown strong positive correlations between the degree of adiposity and fasting triglycerides, even after correcting for age and other variables [10,12]. In the LRC Prevalence Study it was the strongest independent correlate of triglyceride levels in both men and women [13]. This probably reflects the association between increases in body weight and increases in VLDL synthesis [12]. Plasma cholesterol is also positively correlated with body

1

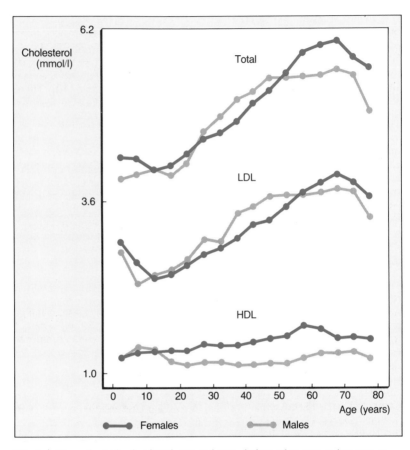

Fig. 1.4. Mean plasma levels of total, LDL and HDL cholesterol in men and women at different ages. Adapted by permission from Schonfeld, *Artery* 1979, 5:305–329.

mass index, although less strongly than triglyceride. This presumably reflects increases in VLDL cholesterol rather than LDL cholesterol, which is independently correlated with body mass index only in young men. HDL cholesterol is inversely correlated with body weight and obesity is a common cause of secondary hypoalphalipoproteinaemia.

Physical activity
Much has been written about the effect of exercise on serum lipids and lipoproteins. Aerobic exercise, such as jogging or cross-country skiing, when performed with sufficient intensity and frequency, results in appreciable reduc-

tions in fasting triglyceride, total and LDL cholesterol, and marked rises in HDL cholesterol. Such differences are even more evident in marathon runners than in joggers. The extent of these changes correlates with the degree of fitness achieved, as gauged by maximal oxygen consumption, and is independent of other influences such as body weight and cigarette consumption. However, dietary factors, including alcohol, may play a role in determining the extent of the rise in HDL cholesterol in runners. The amount of exercise required to influence lipoprotein levels is considerable, equivalent to running 10 miles/week for 6–12 months [14].

The reduction in triglyceride levels with exercise has been attributed to an increased rate of removal consequent on increases in lipoprotein lipase in muscle and adipose tissue. This could also explain the increase in HDL cholesterol, which is mainly HDL_2, in that during lipolysis of triglyceride-rich lipoproteins surface components including free cholesterol are released into plasma. Uptake of the latter by HDL_3 and the subsequent action of LCAT would result, it has been postulated, in an increased rate of formation of HDL_2. An alternative explanation is provided by the observation that hepatic lipase levels are decreased by physical training, one action of this enzyme being to promote conversion of HDL_2 back to HDL_3.

Influence of diet and other habits

A vast literature exists on the influence of dietary factors on serum lipids, reflecting both the importance and complexity of the subject. We will attempt to summarize the main effects of the major constituents of diets commonly eaten in Europe and North America. The burgeoning topic of fish-oil will be dealt with separately in a subsequent chapter.

Calories

Caloric excess sufficient to cause obesity is probably the commonest cause of fasting hypertriglyceridaemia and is due to an increase in VLDL. One possible mechanism is that expanded adipocytes are relatively insulin-resistant and that this results in reactive hyperinsulinism, which leads to stimulation of hepatic triglyceride synthesis and thus to an increased rate of secretion of VLDL. Alternatively, triglyceride clearance may be defective, resulting in a reduced rate of catabolism of VLDL in peripheral tissues. Whatever the mechanism, reduction of body weight to within the desirable range for height, build and sex by restricting caloric intake will often bring serum triglycerides down to within the normal range. Caloric restriction sufficient to induce weight reduction causes a rise in HDL cholesterol in obese individuals, in whom levels tend to be low.

Carbohydrates

Some hypertriglyceridaemic subjects exhibit the phenomenon of carbohydrate-induction in that their serum triglycerides rise even more on carbohydrate-rich diets. This rise is accompanied by increases in plasma insulin levels, and in the size and triglyceride:protein ratio of VLDL parti-

1

cles. The latter phenomena are suggestive of increased triglyceride synthesis. However, some studies have shown impaired triglyceride clearance during carbohydrate induction. Since the activity of extrahepatic lipoprotein lipase, which mediates triglyceride clearance, is markedly influenced by insulin, this has led to the suggestion that carbohydrate-induced hypertriglyceridaemia results from defective lipolysis of VLDL, secondary to insulin resistance at the adipocyte level, rather than from an increase in hepatic triglyceride synthesis. Some normal subjects increase their serum triglycerides when fed a carbohydrate-rich diet, especially if this contains a lot of sucrose, but this rise is transient if the diet is isocaloric. Complex carbohydrates, such as starch, have a lesser tendency than sucrose to provoke hypertriglyceridaemia. HDL levels decrease on carbohydrate-rich diets, probably because of an increased rate of catabolism, and LDL levels tend to vary reciprocally with changes in VLDL.

Fat
The fatty acid composition of food is often described in terms of the P : S ratio, that is to say the relative amount of polyunsaturated and saturated fatty acids contained therein. In general, meat and dairy products have low P : S ratios whereas most fish and vegetable sources of fat have high P : S ratios. A notable exception is coconut oil, which has a P : S ratio of 0.02, even less than that of butter, and is used extensively in products labelled as containing 'non-milk fat' or 'vegetable fat'. Margarines differ markedly in respect of P : S ratio, from 0.13 for a hard variety to 2.00 for a soft margarine. The P : S ratio of cooking fats varies from 0.32 for lard to 4.82 for corn oil. Together with milk and cream these 'visible' fats may constitute up to 50% of the fat consumed in the diet and are thus a major determinant of its overall P : S ratio.

In general terms, saturated fats raise the serum cholesterol and polyunsaturated fats cause it to decrease. Similar changes occur in fasting serum triglycerides. Keys *et al.* [15] proposed that the effect of altering the fat content of the diet on the mean serum cholesterol concentration of groups of normal subjects could be estimated (in mg/dl) by applying the equation $2.7S - 1.3P$ to each diet and then calculating the difference, S being the percentage of total calories derived from saturated fat and P the percentage from polyunsaturated fat. Therefore, reducing the saturated fat intake by a given amount has a cholesterol-lowering effect roughly equivalent to supplementing the diet with twice that amount of polyunsaturated fat.

Originally it was thought that monounsaturated fats were neutral in their effect on serum cholesterol and they were ignored in the Keys equation. However, it has now been shown that a diet containing 40% of its calories as monounsaturated fat, mainly as oleate, lowers LDL cholesterol to a similar extent as a diet containing 40% polyunsaturated fat, mainly as linoleate, and does so without the undesirable reduction in HDL cholesterol which accompanied ingestion of the latter. Furthermore, there was no rise in serum triglyceride on the monounsaturated fat-rich diet such as is observed when low-fat, high-carbohydrate diets are taken [16]. These findings help explain the relatively low serum lipids of populations living in the Mediterranean, whose consumption of olive oil is considerable.

1

Changes in serum cholesterol induced by dietary fat are chiefly due to changes in LDL cholesterol concentration, although iso-directional changes in VLDL cholesterol are a contributory factor. Turnover studies suggest that LDL synthesis is reduced and fractional catabolism enhanced when poly-unsaturated fat is substituted for saturated fat, both effects contributing to a reduction in the size of the intravascular pool of LDL. These changes are accompanied by alterations in the fatty acid composition of the lipid con-stituents of VLDL and LDL, with an increase in the linoleic:oleic acid ratio of cholesterol esters, and by a transient increase in the faecal excretion of neutral sterols and bile acids. The decrease in serum cholesterol induced by polyunsaturated fat feeding in normal subjects can be accounted for by this increase in cholesterol excretion. The effects of polyunsaturated fats on HDL have been less well studied but feeding a very high P:S ratio diet has been reported to cause a substantial decrease in its rate of synthesis.

Cholesterol
Changing the amount of cholesterol in the diet influences serum cholesterol to a much lesser extent than does changing the P:S ratio. This was borne out by a study where normal subjects consumed an extra egg per day for 3 months, which increased their daily intake of cholesterol from 300 to 550 mg but had no effect on total serum cholesterol. However, other studies showed that increasing the intake of dietary cholesterol in a similar manner resulted in a significant increase in LDL cholesterol. Interestingly, cholesterol ingested in the form of shellfish has relatively little effect on serum cholesterol in nor-mal subjects [17]. One of the main difficulties in assessing the importance of dietary cholesterol is the considerable variability of response between in-dividuals. Apart from its source the effect of dietary cholesterol is influenced by the P:S ratio of the accompanying triglyceride, as shown in Fig. 1.5.

Protein
Several studies have shown that substituting soya bean protein for animal protein in the diet results in a fall in serum cholesterol, despite the fat and cholesterol content of the diet being kept constant. The mechanism of this effect is uncertain but the observation itself might explain why some popu-lations in the Far East, where animal protein intake is less than in the West, have lower serum cholesterol levels than would be expected from calcula-tions based solely on the fat and cholesterol content of their diet. Vegetarians are known to have lower serum lipids than non-vegetarians but this is only partly attributable to the source of protein, in view of the high P:S ratio and low cholesterol content of vegetarian diets. HDL cholesterol levels tend to be lower in vegetarians than in subjects on normal diets but their HDL:total cholesterol ratios are higher.

Fibre
Cellulose has no cholesterol-lowering effect but pectin, oat-bran and guar cause a modest decrease when given in very large amounts. Addition of mixed

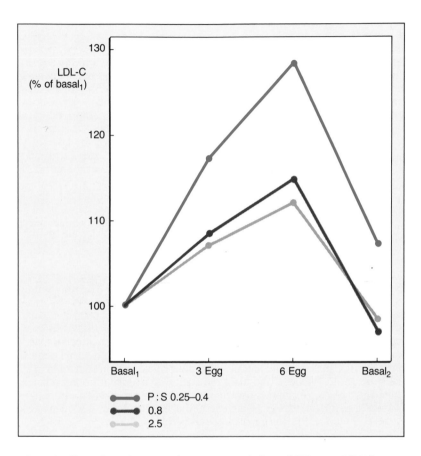

Fig. 1.5. Effects of supplementing diets containing cholesterol 300 mg and 40% fat, of P:S ratios 0.25–0.4, 0.8 or 2.5, with three eggs (cholesterol 750 mg) and six eggs (cholesterol 1500 mg) on LDL cholesterol, expressed as a percentage of the basal values. Adapted by permission from Schonfeld *et al.*, *J Clin Invest* 1982, 69:1072–1080. © American Society for Clinical Investigation.

fibre to the diet can increase faecal neutral sterol excretion but has no effect on serum cholesterol. Thus, under normal circumstances much of the cholesterol-lowering effect of dietary fibre can probably be explained by its having replaced some of the saturated fat in the diet.

Alcohol
Regular consumption of alcohol leads to appreciable increases in HDL cholesterol, an effect which is independent of all other variables. People drinking

two units per day in the Cooperative Lipoprotein Phenotyping Study had HDL cholesterol levels which were 0.33 mmol/l higher than non-drinkers [18]. The increase in HDL involves both HDL_2 and HDL_3 and may reflect an alcohol-induced increase in lipoprotein lipase. There is also an association between alcohol and serum triglyceride levels, although the correlation is much weaker than for HDL cholesterol and disappeared in one study when allowance was made for tobacco consumption [12]. In contrast to these positive correlations LDL cholesterol tends to be negatively correlated with alcohol intake.

Coffee
A number of surveys have shown that ingestion of large quantities of coffee, especially boiled coffee, is associated with a rise in serum cholesterol. This effect is not observed when equivalent quantities of tea are drunk nor with instant coffee and is therefore unlikely to be due to caffeine. A recent review of the evidence concluded that under normal circumstances the cholesterol-raising effect of coffee can probably be ignored but that this does not neces-sarily apply to hypercholesterolaemic individuals, especially those with a high intake [19].

Tobacco
Cigarette smokers in the Framingham Offspring Study had HDL cholesterol levels which were significantly lower than non-smokers or ex-smokers of more than one year's duration. Studies of the mechanism involved suggest that smoking impairs lipolysis and prevents the postprandial increase in HDL_2 normally seen in non-smokers after a fatty meal. This explanation is supported by the independent correlation observed between smoking and plasma triglycerides.

Influence of intercurrent disease

Severe metabolic traumas such as myocardial infarction or an acute viral ill-ness have been shown markedly to affect serum lipids. The most obvious change after a myocardial infarct is a fall in total cholesterol, mainly reflecting a decrease in LDL, as illustrated in Fig. 1.6. This is accompanied by a rise in plasma triglyceride, presumably catecholamine and corticosteroid-mediated, and by a slight fall in HDL cholesterol. These changes are not apparent until 24 hours after the onset of the event but once established may take 6–12 weeks to resolve completely. Similar changes accompany surgical operations or febrile illnesses.

The well documented inverse correlation between serum cholesterol and cancer is thought to be mainly a reflection of the persistent reduction in serum cholesterol which results from the presence of a neoplasm, sometimes occult.

Seasonal and day-to-day variation

Intraindividual variation reflects both analytical imprecision and biological variability. In normal subjects variations in fasting serum lipids over the

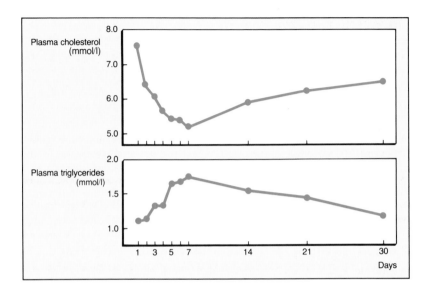

Fig. 1.6. Changes in plasma cholesterol and triglyceride over 30 days in 15 patients after a myocardial infarct. Adapted by permission from Avogaro *et al.*, *Eur J Clin Invest* 1978, 8:121–129.

course of one year ranged from 4 to 11% for total cholesterol, 13 to 41% for triglyceride and 4 to 12% for HDL cholesterol. Over 60% of these variations were attributed to biological fluctuations, the remainder to analytical variability [20]. Part of the biological fluctuation may be explained by seasonal changes in that there is a tendency for total cholesterol and triglyceride to fall during the summer and for HDL cholesterol to rise. Seasonal swings appear to be either light- or temperature-related, being most marked in those parts of the world which show the greatest differential in these respects between winter and summer. In women there is a suggestion that the menstrual cycle may influence serum lipids, with a tendency for cholesterol and triglyceride levels to be higher and HDL cholesterol to be lower during the follicular phase than during the luteal phase. Presumably these differences are related to changes in oestrogen levels, which peak just prior to ovulation. However, the degree of variation observed is relatively small and results of separate studies have sometimes been inconsistent. Although some of the biological variation in plasma lipids reflects changes in factors such as body weight, diet and exercise, much of it remains unexplained. However, its undoubted existence emphasizes the need to obtain multiple samples before diagnosing hyperlipidaemia in an individual.

Annotated references   1

1. GURR MI, JAMES AT: *Lipid Biochemistry: An Introduction.* London: Chapman and Hall, 1971.
A fact-packed paperback on the biochemistry of lipid metabolism.

2. MASORO EJ: *Physiological Chemistry of Lipids in Mammals.* Philadelphia: W.B. Saunders, 1968.
A readable and detailed account of the physics and biochemistry of mammalian lipids of physiological importance.

3. PRESS M, KIKUCHI H, SHIMOYAMA T, THOMPSON GR: **Diagnosis and treatment of essential fatty acid deficiency in man.** *Br Med J* 1974, 2:247–250.
A description of the clinical and diagnostic features of essential fatty acid deficiency in three patients with malabsorption due to intestinal resection.

4. JACKSON RL, GOTTO AM: **Phospholipids in biology and medicine.** *N Engl J Med* 1974, 290:24–29 and 87–93.
A brief review of the role of phospholipids in membranes, lipoproteins and the coagulation pathway.

5. GOODMAN DS, NOBLE RO, DELL RB: **Three-pool model of the long-term turnover of plasma cholesterol in man.** *J Lipid Res* 1973, 14:178–188.
A classic paper describing the mathematical model which best fits the data obtained in very long-term studies of cholesterol turnover.

6. GRUNDY SM, AHRENS EH, DAVIGNON J: **The interaction of cholesterol absorption and cholesterol synthesis in man.** *J Lipid Res* 1969, 10:304–315.
Cholesterol balance studies designed to examine the effects of dietary cholesterol in regulating endogenous cholesterol synthesis.

7. THOMPSON GR: **Plasma lipids and lipoproteins, and the hyperlipoproteinaemias.** In *Biochemical Aspects of Human Disease* edited by Elkeles RS, Tavill AS. Oxford: Blackwell, 1983, pp 85–123.
An up-to-date account of the pathophysiology of plasma lipoproteins.

8. TAMIR I, HEISS G, GLUECK CJ, CHRISTENSEN B, KWITEROVICH P, RIFKIND BM: **Lipid and lipoprotein distributions in white children ages 6–19 years. The Lipid Research Clinics Program Prevalence Study.** *J Clin Dis* 1981, 34:27–39.
Useful data from the LRC Prevalence Study on the distribution of plasma lipids and lipoproteins in children and adolescents in North America.

9. HEISS G, TAMIR I, DAVIS CE, TYROLER HA, RIFKIND BM, SCHONFELD G, JACOBS D, FRANTZ ID: **Lipoprotein cholesterol distributions in selected North American populations: the Lipid Research Clinics Program Prevalence Study.** *Circulation* 1980, 61:302–315.
Data on the concentration of cholesterol in VLDL, LDL and HDL in a subset of men and women aged 20–59 in the LRC Prevalence Study, including changes with age, sex differences and effects of hormone therapy in females.

10.   CONNOR SL, CONNOR WE, SEXTON G, CALVIN L, BACON S: The effects of age, body weight and family relationships on plasma lipoproteins and lipids in men, women and children of randomly selected families. *Circulation* 1982, 65:1290–1298.

An investigation into the role of genetic versus environmental influences in determining intrafamilial trends in plasma lipids and lipoproteins.

11.   GREEN MS, HEISS G, RIFKIND BM, COOPER GR, WILLIAMS OD, TYROLER HA: The ratio of plasma high density lipoprotein cholesterol to total and low density lipoprotein cholesterol: age-related changes and race and sex differences in selected North American populations: the Lipid Research Clinics Program Prevalence Study. *Circulation* 1985, 72:93–104.

Another useful contribution from the LRC Prevalence Study; this one examines the influence of age, race and sex on HDL: total and HDL: LDL cholesterol ratios.

12.   PHILLIPS NR, HAVEL RJ, KANE JP: Levels and interrelationships of serum and lipoprotein cholesterol and triglycerides. Association with adiposity and the consumption of ethanol, tobacco and beverages containing caffeine. *Arteriosclerosis* 1981, 1:13–24.

A San Francisco account of the role of various physiological and environmental factors in determining serum lipids and lipoproteins.

13.   COWAN LD, WILCOSKY T, CRIQUI MH, BARRETT-CONNOR E, SUCHINDRAM CM, WALLACE R, LASKARZEWSKI P, WALDEN C: Demographic, behavioural, biochemical and dietary correlates of plasma triglycerides. Lipid Research Clinics Program Prevalence Study. *Arteriosclerosis* 1985, 5:466–480.

More data from the LRC Prevalence Study, here dealing with factors influencing the concentration of plasma triglyceride.

14.   WILLIAMS PT, WOOD PD, HASKELL WL, VRANIZAN K: The effects of running mileage and duration on plasma lipoprotein levels. *JAMA* 1982, 247:2674–2679.

A year-long study of the effects of regular exercise on fitness, body weight and plasma lipoproteins in middle-aged men.

15.   KEYS A, ANDERSON JT, GRANDE F: Serum cholesterol response to changes in the diet. 1. Iodine value of dietary fat versus 2S – P. *Metabolism* 1965, 14:747–758.

A much quoted but probably erroneous equation which relates the fatty acid composition of the diet to changes in serum cholesterol (see [16]).

16.   GRUNDY SM: Comparison of monounsaturated fatty acids and carbohydrates for lowering plasma cholesterol. *N Engl J Med* 1986, 314:745–748.

This paper points out that dietary monounsaturated fatty acids lower LDL cholesterol despite their having been regarded previously as neutral in this respect and on this account omitted from the Keys formula.

17.   CONNOR WE, LIN DS: The effect of shellfish in the diet upon the plasma lipid level in humans. *Metabolism* 1982, 31:1046–1051.

Some shellfish contain only cholesterol whereas others also contain other sterols, which competitively inhibit cholesterol absorption and thus minimize changes in serum cholesterol when ingested.

18. CASTELLI WP, DOYLE JT, GORDON T, HAMES CG, HJORTLAND M, HULLEY SB, KAGAN A, ZUKEL WJ: **Alcohol and blood lipids.** *Lancet* 1977, ii:153–155.
A heartening analysis which illustrates that a little of what-you-fancy does you good, with respect to alcohol and HDL.

19. THELLE DS, HEYDEN S, FODOR JG: **Coffee and cholesterol in epidemiological and experimental studies.** *Atherosclerosis* 1987, 67:97–103.
Too much coffee, if boiled in Scandinavian style, can aggravate hypercholesterolaemia but reasonable quantities of filtered or instant coffee seem relatively harmless.

20. DEMACKER PNM, SCHADE RWB, JANSEN RTP, VAN'T LAAR A: **Intra-individual variation of serum cholesterol, triglycerides and high density lipoprotein cholesterol in normal humans.** *Atherosclerosis* 1982, 45:259–266.
A careful study of the sources of variation which account for the quite marked fluctuations in serum lipids observed when these were measured repeatedly over the course of a year.

1

2 LIPOPROTEIN METABOLISM

Apolipoproteins

Introduction

Before describing the metabolism of the various lipoprotein classes it is necessary to review briefly their physical properties and those of their constituent apolipoproteins. Plasma lipoproteins differ according to flotation rate (S_f), hydrated density (d), size and electrophoretic mobility, as summarized in Table 2.1. Currently, the most popular classification is that based on differences in density, which are used to separate them in the ultracentrifuge, rather than

2

on electrophoretic mobility. Lipoproteins also differ importantly in respect of their content of apolipoproteins or apoproteins, as shown in Table 2.2.

Table 2.1. Physical properties of plasma lipoproteins.

	Density (g/ml)	Flotation rate $S_f 1.063$	Flotation rate $S_f 1.20$	Mean diameter (nm)	Electro- phoretic mobility
Chylomicrons	<0.95	>400		100–1000	origin
VLDL	<1.006	20–400		43	preβ
IDL	1.006–1.019	12–20		27 ⎫	
LDL	1.019–1.063	0–12		22 ⎬	β
HDL$_2$	1.063–1.125		3.5–9.0	9.5 ⎫	
HDL$_3$	1.125–1.21		0–3.5	6.5 ⎭	α
Lp(a)	1.051–1.082		≅24	26	preβ$_1$

Table 2.2. Protein composition of lipoproteins in fasting plasma.

	Chylomicrons	VLDL	LDL	HDL
Total protein (mg/dl plasma)	—	6*	80*	190*
Apoproteins (% of total protein)				
ApoA-I	Tr	Tr	Tr	66*
ApoA-II	Tr	Tr	Tr	20*
ApoB	5–20	37	97*	—
ApoC-I	15	3	Tr	3*
ApoC-II	15	7	Tr	Tr
ApoC-III	40–50	40	2*	4*
ApoD	—	—	—	5*
ApoE	4	13	1*	1*

*From Gotto *et al.* [5].

Main functions

Apoproteins have three main functions: they help solubilize cholesterol esters and triglyceride by interacting with phospholipids; they regulate the reaction of these lipids with enzymes such as LCAT, lipoprotein lipase and hepatic lipase, and they bind to cell surface receptors and thus determine the sites of uptake and rates of degradation of other lipoprotein constituents, notably cholesterol. The mechanism by which apoproteins bind lipids is dependent primarily upon hydrophobic bonding between the fatty acyl chains of phospholipids and the non-polar regions of apoproteins, with ionic interaction between the polar head groups of phospholipids and pairs of oppositely charged amino acids in the α-helical regions of the apoprotein playing a secondary, stabilizing role. Lipid protein interaction has a reciprocal quality in that, whereas apoproteins effect the water-solubilization of lipids, the latter enhance the solubility of apoproteins by preventing aggregation between adjacent polypeptide chains.

2

Structure

Individual apoproteins used to be designated on the basis of their carboxy-terminal amino acids but this nomenclature has now been superseded by the alphabetical terminology introduced by Alaupovic [1].

Apolipoprotein A

Apolipoprotein A is the chief protein constituent of HDL and is subdivided into apoA-I and apoA-II. Both these apoproteins have glutamine as their carboxy-terminal amino acid. The molecular weight of apoA-I is 28 300 and of apoA-II is 17 000, the latter consisting in humans of two identical polypeptide chains linked by a disulphide bond. There is some evidence that when the two apoproteins exist together, as in HDL, apoA-II enhances the lipid binding properties of apoA-I, possibly by dint of protein-protein interaction. Another function of apoA-I is to activate LCAT.

Apolipoprotein B

Apolipoprotein B or apoB is heterogeneous; $apoB_{100}$, with a molecular weight of 512 000, is found mainly in chylomicrons, VLDL and LDL whereas $apoB_{48}$, with a molecular weight of 241 000, is found only in chylomicrons. ApoB is extremely insoluble in water in the delipidated state, and this has been a major obstacle to determining its primary structure. However, by cloning the gene, the amino acid sequence of both forms of apoB has now been deduced, together with the fact that $apoB_{48}$ represents the amino-terminal half of $apoB_{100}$. The synthesis of two proteins from one gene appears to be brought about by the insertion of a stop codon into messenger RNA during or after transcription in the intestine but not the liver [2]. $ApoB_{100}$ is a ligand for the LDL receptor but $apoB_{48}$ is not.

Apolipoprotein C

Apolipoprotein C comprises at least three distinct apoproteins, which occur as major constituents of VLDL and minor constituents of HDL. ApoC-I is a single polypeptide chain with a molecular weight of 6631, apoC-II has a molecular weight of 8837 and apoC-III has a molecular weight of 8764 and exists in three forms according to whether the molecule has 0, 1 or 2 sialic acid residues in its carbohydrate moiety. ApoC-II is an activator of lipoprotein lipase.

Apolipoprotein E

Apolipoprotein E (apoE) is found in VLDL, IDL and HDL, entering plasma mainly in the form of nascent HDL. It is polymorphic, with a molecular weight of around 34 000, and its carboxy-terminal is alanine. It serves several functions, including the receptor-mediated transfer of cholesterol between tissues and plasma [3].

Other apoproteins

Other apoproteins which require mention are apoD, a minor constituent of HDL; apoA-IV, a component of intestinal chylomicrons; and apo(a), one of the protein constituents of the Lp(a) lipoprotein. Detailed reviews of apoprotein structure and function have been published recently by Mahley *et al.* [4] and Gotto *et al.* [5]. The chromosomal location of the genes encoding all the major apoproteins is shown in Fig. 2.1.

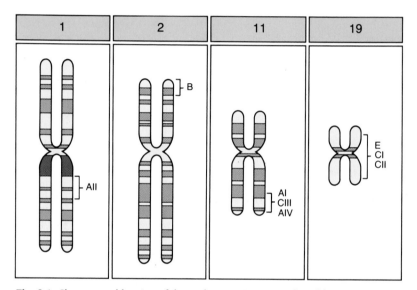

Fig. 2.1. Chromosomal location of the apolipoprotein genes. Adapted by permission from Breslow, Lipoprotein genetics and molecular biology. In *Plasma Lipoproteins* edited by Gotto. Amsterdam: Elsevier, 1987, pp 359–397.

Lipoproteins

Chylomicrons

Chylomicrons are the largest lipoprotein particles, varying in size from 100 to 1000 nm, and consist mainly of triglyceride, together with lesser amounts of phospholipid, free cholesterol, cholesterol esters and protein. They are the form in which most of the dietary triglyceride is transported from its intestinal site of absorption into the systemic circulation. Peak chylomicronaemia normally occurs between 3 and 6 hours after ingestion of a fatty meal, and then gradually declines. The rate of removal of chylomicrons from plasma is rapid, with a half-life of less than 1 hour, and normally they are undetectable after a 12-hour fast.

2

Protein is a relatively minor constituent of chylomicrons (1–2%) but plays a major functional role. This applies especially to apoB$_{48}$, as illustrated by the complete absence of chylomicrons from the plasma of patients with aβ-lipoproteinaemia, in whom there is an inherited defect of apoB synthesis. Approximately 5–20% of the protein of lymph chylomicrons is apoB$_{48}$, the remainder consisting of apoA and apoC (Table 2.2). Lymph chylomicrons lose apoA but gain apoC and E from HDL when they enter plasma and it has been suggested that virtually all their content of apoC is obtained in this manner.

VLDL (preβ-lipoprotein)

In structure and composition VLDL are similar to chylomicrons but are smaller, ranging in size from 25 to 100 nm, and contain less triglyceride but more cholesterol, phospholipid and protein. The protein consists of a mixture of apoC, apoE and apoB$_{100}$ (Table 2.2), the latter's essential role being illustrated by absence of VLDL, as well as chylomicrons, from the plasma of patients with aβ-lipoproteinaemia.

The main differences between chylomicrons and VLDL are their sites of synthesis and the source of the triglyceride being transported. VLDL are mainly synthesized in the liver and their chief function is the transport of endogenously synthesized triglyceride. However, some VLDL are synthesized in the small intestine, where they act as a vehicle for the reabsorption of endogenous cholesterol and fatty acids of biliary origin.

VLDL synthesis is promoted by an increase in the flux of FFA to the liver and also in situations attended by an increase in the rate of hepatic synthesis of endogenous fatty acids, as occurs during a period of high carbohydrate intake. Enhanced synthesis of VLDL triglyceride is accompanied by an increased incorporation of labelled amino acids into VLDL protein, predominantly into apoB rather than apoC; this suggests that, like chylomicrons, VLDL probably acquire much of their apoC from HDL after their entry into plasma. The rate of turnover of VLDL in humans is less rapid than that of chylomicrons, with a half-life of 2–4 hours.

VLDL particles show a considerable variation in size, smaller particles having a lower ratio of apoC : apoB than larger ones. Subsequent lipolysis renders these particles even smaller and they are then referred to as VLDL remnants or IDL, this term indicating their role as intermediates in the conversion of a VLDL particle to an LDL particle. There is evidence that a greater proportion of small VLDL particles (S$_f$ 20–60) are converted into LDL via IDL as compared with large VLDL (S$_f$ 60–400), which are converted to a form of

2

IDL which is removed from plasma before undergoing conversion to LDL [6]. Carbohydrate-induced hypertriglyceridaemia is characterized by an increase in not only the number but also the size of the VLDL particles released into plasma, which may explain the reciprocal fall in LDL cholesterol which this engenders.

IDL

The term IDL as used here refers specifically to the intermediate particles formed during conversion of VLDL to LDL, sometimes termed VLDL remnants, as distinct from chylomicron remnants. Operationally they are isolated from fasting plasma by preparative ultracentrifugation at d 1.006–1.019 or by zonal ultracentrifugation. Using the latter technique the concentration of IDL in normal subjects has been shown to be one-tenth that of LDL, with a composition between that of VLDL and LDL (see Table 1.1) and exhibiting slow preβ mobility on agarose gel. As discussed later, accumulation of IDL in familial hypercholesterolaemia (FH) suggests that it is normally cleared by the LDL receptor, although it is uncertain whether it is the apoB or apoE on the surface of IDL which acts as the ligand.

LDL (β-lipoprotein)

LDL is the major cholesterol-carrying particle in plasma and differs from its precursor VLDL in its much lower triglyceride content and in retaining only one of the various apoproteins found in VLDL, namely apoB$_{100}$. LDL shows some variation in particle size and composition and can be separated by density gradient ultracentrifugation into two major subfractions, light and heavy LDL, the former being a precursor of the latter [7]. However, the absolute amount of apoB per LDL particle is remarkably constant and similar to that in VLDL. This suggests that each LDL particle is derived from the catabolism of a single VLDL particle [8]. Turnover studies suggest that the rate of turnover of VLDL-apoB can account for all the LDL-apoB synthesized, except in FH where direct secretion of LDL sometimes occurs [9]. However, in most circumstances LDL synthesis equals the product of the rate of VLDL synthesis and the percentage of VLDL converted into LDL.

Apart from the synthetic rate, the other major determinant of LDL concentration in plasma is the rate at which it is catabolized. Normally the fractional catabolic rate of LDL-apoB is in the region of 0.3–0.4, that is to say 30–40% of the intravascular pool is catabolized per day, of which around half is via the receptor-mediated pathway (see LDL receptor). Both environmental and genetic factors influence this aspect of LDL metabolism, such as the type of dietary fat eaten and mutations of the LDL receptor and apoB genes.

HDL (α-lipoprotein)

HDL is subdivided into HDL_2 and HDL_3, the former being isolated between d 1.063 and 1.125, the latter between d 1.125 and 1.21. Both have α-mobility on electrophoresis but HDL_2 contains less protein than HDL_3 and is present in plasma in smaller amounts.

2

Over 90% of the protein in HDL is apoA, the ratio of apoA-I : apoA-II being 3 : 1 in both HDL_2 and HDL_3. Although only 3–5% of HDL_2 protein and 1–2% of HDL_3 protein is apoC, nevertheless roughly half of the apoC in fasting plasma is found in HDL. Studies with labelled VLDL have shown that apoC rapidly transfers from VLDL to HDL and vice versa. Thus HDL appears to act as a reservoir for apoC derived from chylomicrons and VLDL during lipolysis, the apoC being picked up again by chylomicrons upon entering the blood via the thoracic duct during alimentary lipaemia. Release of surface components from triglyceride-rich lipoproteins during lipolysis promotes conversion of HDL_3 to HDL_2.

Recent technological advances have added further subclasses of HDL to our knowledge. Gradient gel electrophoresis, which separates proteins according to size, enables at least five HDL subclasses to be defined. On immunochromatography two distinct groups of HDL particles appear to exist in human plasma, those containing both apoA-I and apoA-II and those having A-I without A-II. The metabolic and clinical implications of these various HDL subclasses are as yet largely unknown.

HDL is synthesized in both the liver and small intestine and in its nascent form appears as bilayered discs on electron microscopy [10]. These nascent particles consist mainly of apoE, apoC, phospholipid and free cholesterol. Subsequently the apoE is largely replaced by apoA-I, most of the cholesterol becomes esterified as a result of the action of the enzyme LCAT in blood and the particle becomes spherical. The dominant role of the liver in the synthesis of apoE and apoC contrasts with the dual origins of apoA-I from liver and small intestine, as shown in Table 2.3. The accumulation of cholesterol esters in the reticulo-endothelial system of patients with HDL deficiency (Tangier disease) suggests that HDL normally plays a major role in the mobilization of tissue cholesterol.

Turnover studies show that about 50% of HDL is located within the intravascular compartment, the half-life of the apoA-I and apoA-II moieties being similar. In general there appears to be a reciprocal relationship between the concentrations of VLDL and HDL in plasma, the decreased level of HDL induced by high carbohydrate diets being due apparently to increased catabolism.

Lp(a)

Although it is a lipoprotein, the concentration of Lp(a) varies in humans from nil to more than 100 mg/dl and its physiological function remains unknown. It is larger but more dense than LDL and exhibits slow preβ mobility on

Table 2.3. Contribution by liver and intestine to plasma apoproteins in the rat.

Apoprotein	% from liver	% from intestine
ApoA-I	44	56
ApoA-IV	41	59
ApoB	85	16
ApoC	95	5
ApoE	99	1

Data from Wu and Windmueller, *J Biol Chem* 1979, 254:7316–7322.

electrophoresis ('sinking preβ' lipoprotein). Its lipid composition is similar to LDL but it has a higher protein content due to the presence of 1 mole of apo(a) per mole of apoB$_{100}$, the two proteins being linked by disulphide bonds [11]. Apo(a) is polymorphic, exhibits close homology with plasminogen and has a high content of carbohydrate. Available data suggest that Lp(a) is derived solely from the liver but not via the VLDL pathway. Despite its content of apoB$_{100}$ there is conflicting evidence as to whether Lp(a) is catabolized via the LDL receptor. *In vitro* it shows a marked tendency to aggregate.

Enzymes, receptors and transfer proteins

Lipoprotein lipases

Intravenous injection of heparin results in the rapid appearance in plasma of lipolytic enzymes, referred to operationally as post-heparin lipolytic activity (PHLA). This activity is composite, reflecting the presence of both triglyceride lipases and phospholipases. The action of heparin is to displace lipolytic enzymes from their sites of attachment to vascular endothelium and a maximum effect is obtained by a dose of 1 mg (100 i.u.) per kg body weight.

PHLA comprises at least two distinct triglyceride lipases. Extrahepatic or lipoprotein lipase is found mainly in adipose tissue and skeletal muscle where it is located on glycosoaminoglycan chains anchored to the luminal surface of the capillary endothelium. It is activated by apoC-II and inhibited by 1 mol sodium chloride and by protamine sulphate. Hepatic lipase is located on the luminal surface of hepatic endothelial cells and is unaffected by the inhibitors and activators of the extrahepatic enzyme. Both enzymes are triglyceride lipases and also possess phospholipase A-like activity, especially hepatic lipase.

These lipases are involved in the catabolism of triglyceride-rich lipoproteins, namely chylomicrons and VLDL. Lipoprotein lipase is the more active of the two in this respect, hydrolysis of triglyceride taking place mainly within capillaries serving adipose tissue and skeletal and cardiac muscle. ApoC-II promotes this process by facilitating binding of chylomicrons and VLDL to the enzyme. The ability of the latter to clear triglyceride is potentially saturable and excessive accumulation of VLDL in plasma can impair chylomicron removal. The relative amounts of lipoprotein lipase in adipose tissue versus muscle is higher in women than men and is correlated with their higher HDL cholesterol levels and lower VLDL concentrations. The amount of enzyme in adipose tissue in men increases during a period of regular consumption of alcohol, whereas regular exercise increases the enzyme content of skeletal muscle, both activities being attended by a rise in HDL cholesterol.

2

The function of hepatic lipase is less well established but it is probably involved in the catabolism of the remnant particles which result from the action of the extrahepatic enzyme on chylomicrons and VLDL. The former process presumably occurs in the liver and involves hydrolysis of most of the residual triglyceride and much of the phospholipid of remnant particles, resulting in the formation of LDL. A second proposed role for hepatic lipase involves conversion of HDL_2 back to HDL_3 by hydrolysis of triglycerides and phospholipids present in HDL_2.

The two enzymes can be separated from each other by heparin-sepharose affinity chromatography and by immunoprecipitation, as discussed in detail elsewhere [12,13].

A simplified scheme of lipoprotein metabolism illustrating the twin pathways whereby triglyceride-rich lipoproteins enter plasma and then undergo conversion into cholesterol-rich lipoproteins as a result of the action of these lipoprotein lipases is shown in Fig. 2.2.

Lecithin : cholesterol acyltransferase

Lecithin : cholesterol acyltransferase or LCAT is an enzyme which originates in the liver but exerts its action in plasma, where it is responsible for transesterifying cholesterol with fatty acids derived from the 2-position of lecithin [14] as shown in Fig. 2.3.

Normally, LCAT activity is detectable in both the high-density and very-high-density (d 1.21–1.25) fractions of plasma, the purified enzyme having a molecular weight of around 60 000 [15]. LCAT activity in plasma can be assayed either with lipoproteins or with an artificial substrate, consisting of a mixture of lecithin and free cholesterol. Under these circumstances its activity has been shown to be enhanced by apoA-I, apoA-IV and apoC-I, whereas apoD appears to exert a stabilizing effect on the enzyme.

LCAT utilizes linoleate in the esterification of cholesterol in preference to the other fatty acids which occur in the 2-position of lecithin. Thus the enrichment of the linoleate content of plasma lecithin which accompanies ingestion of a polyunsaturated fat diet leads to an increase in the proportion of cholesterol linoleate in plasma. The physiological substrate for LCAT has been suggested to be HDL_3. The latter's high phospholipid content enables it to act as

2

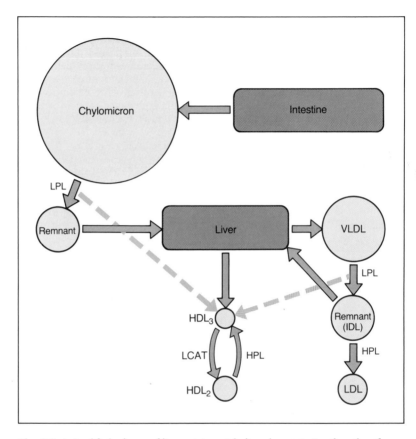

Fig. 2.2. A simplified scheme of lipoprotein metabolism demonstrating the roles of lipoprotein lipase (LPL) and hepatic lipase (HPL) in the conversion of triglyceride-rich chylomicrons and VLDL into cholesterol-rich HDL and LDL. The broken lines represent surface components of chylomicrons and VLDL released during lipolysis.

an efficient acceptor of free cholesterol, including that in cell membranes, and the presence of apoA-I promotes subsequent esterification by LCAT. Thus, the mature HDL_2 particle contains mainly esterified cholesterol which is then transported to the liver to undergo catabolism. The free cholesterol of VLDL and LDL can also serve as a substrate for LCAT. The enzyme also plays a role in the catabolism of triglyceride-rich particles, by simultaneously removing free cholesterol and lecithin in equimolar amounts from their surface while their core lipids are reduced by the action of triglyceride lipases.

Methods for isolating and quantitating LCAT are described in detail elsewhere [15].

2

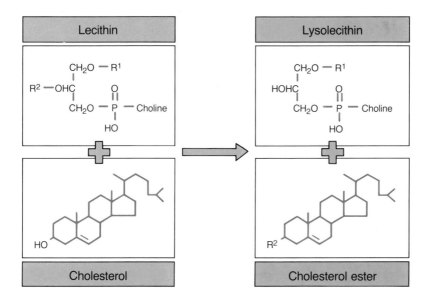

Fig. 2.3. The LCAT reaction. In human plasma the fatty acid in the 2-position of lecithin (R^2) is either mono- or polyunsaturated. From [14].

LDL receptor

A series of studies from 1973 onwards led to the award in 1985 of the Nobel Prize to Brown and Goldstein for their discovery of the LDL receptor and the cause of FH. A detailed review of the structure–function relationships and genetic determinants of the LDL receptor in particular and of receptor-mediated endocytosis in general was published by these authors in that same year [16] and more recently in an abbreviated form [17].

Their earlier studies showed that cultured skin fibroblasts from normal subjects possess specific cell surface receptors which recognize both $apoB_{100}$ and apoE (B,E receptors) and thereby bind LDL by means of a high-affinity, saturable mechanism. The bound LDL is incorporated into the fibroblast within endocytic vesicles, derived from clathrin-coated pits in which LDL receptors localize on the cell surface. After shedding their coats the endocytic vesicles fuse to become endosomes within which the LDL dissociates from its receptor. The latter recycles to the surface and reenters another coated pit whereas the LDL undergoes lysosomal digestion. This results in degradation of apoB and hydrolysis of cholesterol esters. The free cholesterol that is released serves to control the rate of cholesterol synthesis within the cell by down-regulating the enzyme HMG CoA reductase. Excess free cholesterol is re-esterified within the cell by ACAT, which preferentially uses oleate for this purpose. The rate of synthesis of LDL receptors is, in turn, regulated by a feedback mechanism linked to the cholesterol content of the cell.

More recent studies reveal that the LDL receptor is a single-chain transmembrane protein with five distinct domains: ligand binding, epidermal growth factor precursor homologous, O-linked sugar-containing, membrane spanning, and cytoplasmic. The ligand-binding domain comprises seven repetitive cysteine-rich negatively charged sequences which interact electrostatically with the arginine and lysine-rich fraction of apoB, whereas the cytoplasmic domain functions to direct the receptor into a coated pit. Receptors are synthesized in ribosomes in the rough endoplasmic reticulum and glycosylated in the Golgi apparatus. Mutations of the gene encoding the LDL receptor, which is located on the short arm of chromosome 19, result in impaired degradation of LDL and thus cause FH.

The chief role of the LDL receptor is to provide a constantly available source of cholesterol throughout the body for cell membrane synthesis and for supplying certain organs which require it as a substrate for their metabolic products, e.g. bile acids, sex hormones, corticosteroids. Thus the liver, gonads and adrenals are well provided with LDL receptors, and the liver, because of its size, is the major site of receptor-mediated LDL catabolism. LDL receptors also bind VLDL remnants or IDL and a subfraction of HDL which contains apoE. A diagrammatic representation of the receptor in action is shown in Fig. 2.4.

HMG CoA reductase

HMG CoA reductase is a 97-kilodalton glycoprotein which is found in the endoplasmic reticulum of all cells possessing the ability to synthesize cholesterol, notably the liver, small intestine, adrenals and gonads. The gene encoding this enzyme is located on chromosome 5. The enzyme catalyses the conversion of HMG CoA to mevalonic acid and its activity is down-regulated by its end-product, cholesterol, and also by metabolites such as 26-hydroxycholesterol. Endogenous cholesterol synthesis is decreased by exposing cells to lipoproteins such as LDL which facilitate delivery of exogenous cholesterol and thus down-regulate the enzyme whereas lipoproteins such as HDL which promote cholesterol efflux have the opposite effect.

The coordinated regulation of LDL receptor expression and HMG CoA reductase activity provides a homeostatic mechanism for ensuring an adequate supply of cholesterol to cells such as hepatocytes which metabolize large amounts each day. Pharmacological agents which competitively inhibit HMG CoA reductase block endogenous cholesterol synthesis and thereby stimulate LDL receptor activity, which results in a reduction in plasma levels of LDL cholesterol. This approach has given rise to a new and powerful class of drugs to treat hypercholesterolaemia, the HMG CoA reductase inhibitors (dealt with in a later chapter).

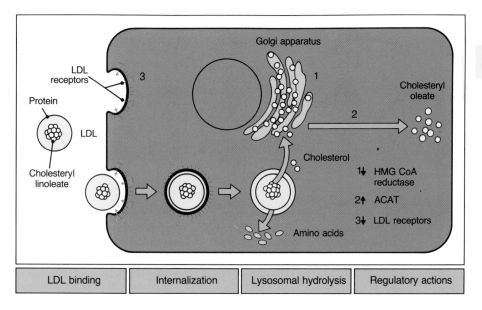

| LDL binding | Internalization | Lysosomal hydrolysis | Regulatory actions |

Fig. 2.4. Diagrammatic representation of a fibroblast showing uptake and partial degradation of LDL via the LDL receptor pathway. The resultant increase in free cholesterol down-regulates HMG CoA reductase and LDL receptor synthesis and results in an increased rate of cholesterol esterification via ACAT. Adapted by permission from Brown and Goldstein, *Proc Natl Acad Sci USA* 1979, 76:3330–3337.

Table 2.4.

Characteristics of hepatic apoB,E receptors
1 Bind lipoproteins containing apoE, $apoB_{100}$ or both
2 Decrease with age and are down-regulated by cholesterol feeding
3 Stimulated by fasting, bile acid deficiency, HMG CoA reductase inhibitors, tri-iodothyrodine and oestrogens
4 Defective in FH

Characteristics of hepatic apoE receptors
1 Bind lipoproteins containing apoE but not $apoB_{100}$
2 Not affected by age or other factors which regulate apoB,E receptors
3 Present in FH

Chylomicron remnant receptor

Chylomicron remnants are removed by a receptor-mediated process in the liver which recognizes the apoE on their surface but not $apoB_{48}$. Evidence that a specific receptor exists and that clearance is not mediated by the B,E or LDL receptor includes observations that chylomicron remnants are cleared normally in patients with homozygous FH, who lack LDL receptors, and that the process responsible is not down-regulated by cholesterol feeding, as is the LDL receptor. Features which distinguish the two types of receptor are listed in Table 2.4.

The identification of apoE as the ligand recognized by the chylomicron remnant receptor stems from observations that lack of apoE, as in apoE deficiency, or the presence of an abnormal isoform, as in type III hyperlipoproteinaemia, leads to accumulation of remnants due to impaired uptake. However, although three apoE-binding proteins have been identified in human liver, none of them possess the necessary cell-surface localization and other properties which would enable them to fulfil the role of a chylomicron remnant receptor [18]. Thus the nature and indeed the existence of the latter remains a matter of conjecture.

Whatever the mechanism, chylomicron remnants are cleared efficiently by the liver, unlike intact chylomicrons, the uptake of which is prevented by their high content of C apoproteins, which are inhibitory in this respect but which decrease during lipolysis.

After binding to liver cells, chylomicron remnants are internalized by endocytosis and, depending upon their content of cholesterol, may down-regulate the LDL receptor. VLDL remnants, in contrast, get taken up by the B,E receptor, as is illustrated by the impaired removal of IDL from plasma seen in FH (Fig. 2.5).

Other lipoprotein receptors

An HDL receptor has been identified in cultured fibroblasts and smooth muscle cells, the expression of which is stimulated by cholesterol loading. HDL_3 is bound more efficiently than HDL_2, and in a reversible manner, this process being accompanied by efflux of free cholesterol from the cell [19]. A hepatic HDL receptor, which recognizes apoA-I, has also been identified and appears to be up-regulated by cholesterol loading in an analogous manner [20]. Whether these two receptors are identical is uncertain nor is it clear to what extent they are involved in irreversible catabolism of HDL, as opposed to simply providing a pathway for reverse cholesterol transport.

Two other lipoprotein receptors have also been described, although it is unclear to what extent they participate in lipoprotein metabolism *in vivo*. The acetyl LDL or scavenger receptor is found in macrophages and hepatic endothelial cells and binds and degrades chemically modified LDL, including acetylated and oxidized LDL. It may well play a key role in atherogenesis in that the amount of native LDL taken up by the B,E receptor on macrophages is insufficient to account for the formation of foam cells whereas uptake of modified LDL by the acetyl LDL receptor, which is unregulated, could provide a plausible explanation for this process.

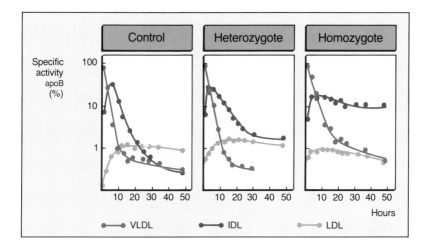

Fig. 2.5. Turnover of ^{125}I-labelled VLDL in a control subject and patients with heterozygous and homozygous FH, respectively. In each instance there is a precursor–product relationship between VLDL and IDL but removal of IDL is delayed in the FH patients, especially the homozygote. Data from Soutar *et al.*, *Atherosclerosis* 1982, 43:217–231.

A β-VLDL receptor has also been identified in macrophages which is specific for chylomicrons, large VLDL particles from hypertriglyceridaemic subjects and the β-migrating VLDL of patients with type III hyperlipoproteinaemia [4].

Lipid transfer proteins

Net movement of cholesterol ester, triglyceride and phospholipids between the various lipoprotein classes in plasma is well recognized, as distinct from the rapid exchange of free cholesterol which also occurs. There is evidence that transfer of cholesterol ester from HDL to VLDL and of triglyceride in the reverse direction is mediated by a protein, sometimes called the cholesterol ester transfer protein (CETP), which is present in the d > 1.25 fraction of plasma. By this means an exit route is provided for cholesterol ester accumulating in HDL as the result of the action of LCAT, thus maintaining continuity of movement of cholesterol from cells into plasma. Absence or deficiency of this factor results in the accumulation of cholesterol ester in HDL.

A second lipid transfer protein has also been identified in the d > 1.25 fraction of plasma which appears to mediate transfer of phospholipids between lipoproteins, including transfer to HDL of lecithin liberated from chylomicrons and VLDL undergoing lipolysis. Methods for isolating and quantifying transfer proteins have been described [21].

2

Metabolic interrelationships between lipoproteins

Lipoprotein metabolism is a dynamic process involving considerable movement of both lipids and apoproteins between the individual classes as well as enzyme-catalysed reactions; these interactions eventually result in receptor-mediated delivery of cholesterol to or its removal from cells. A much simplified scheme which attempts to show these complex relationships is shown in Fig. 2.6. This scheme focuses on the fate of the relatively small amounts of cholesterol transported in plasma but ignores the much greater quantities of triglyceride undergoing disposal by similar pathways. Nevertheless, it provides a useful point of reference to the mechanisms underlying certain forms of hyperlipidaemia, as will become apparent in later chapters.

Annotated references

1. ALAUPOVIC P: **Apolipoproteins and lipoproteins.** *Atherosclerosis* 1971, **13**:141.
An editorial describing the relatively simple alphabetical designation of apolipoproteins which displaced the previously confused and complicated system based on amino-terminal groups.

2. SCOTT J, WALLIS SC, PEASE RJ, KNOTT TJ, POWELL L: **Apolipoprotein B: a novel mechanism for deriving two proteins from one gene.** In *Hyperlipidaemia and Atherosclerosis* edited by Suckling KE, Groot PHE. London: Academic Press, 1988, pp 47–64.
A detailed review of the molecular events which enable the apoB gene to give rise to different forms of apoB, depending upon whether transcription takes place in the liver or small intestine.

3. MAHLEY RW: **Apolipoprotein E: cholesterol transport protein with expanding role in cell biology.** *Science* 1988, **240**:622-630.
A detailed review of a ubiquitous apoprotein with a wide range of actions, including transport of cholesterol within the central nervous system.

4. MAHLEY RW, INNERARITY TL, RALL SC, WEISGRABER KH: **Plasma lipoproteins: apolipoprotein structure and function.** *J Lipid Res* 1984, **25**:1277–1294.
A good general review of apoprotein structure and function which includes the amino acid sequences of all the major apoproteins except apoB.

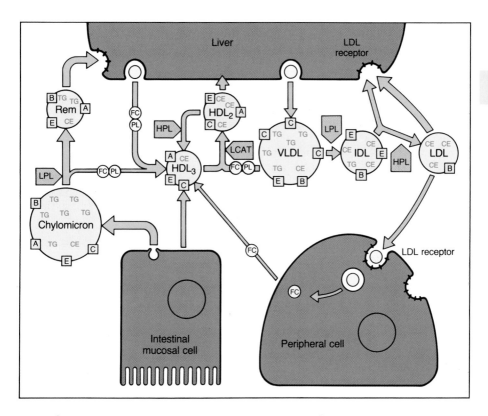

Fig. 2.6. Diagrammatic representation of tissue sites of origin and degradation and the intravascular metabolism of the different lipoprotein classes. A, B, C and E refer to the corresponding apoproteins and FC, PL, CE and TG to free cholesterol, phospholipid, cholesterol ester, and triglyceride, respectively. Chylomicrons transport dietary lipids via lymph into plasma and then get degraded to remnants (Rem) by extrahepatic lipoprotein lipase (LPL), which is activated by apoC-II. Chylomicron remnants are then taken up by hepatic receptors which recognize the apoE on their surface. VLDL carry endogenously synthesized triglyceride from the liver into plasma where, like chylomicrons, they undergo partial degradation to VLDL remnants or IDL. The latter are then either taken up by the LDL receptor, which recognizes both the apoE and the apoB$_{100}$ which they contain (as distinct from the smaller apoB$_{48}$ present in chylomicrons), or are further degraded to LDL, which contains apoB$_{100}$ but not apoE. Hepatic lipase (HPL) may be involved in this process. LDL in turn undergoes catabolism via at least two major pathways, one of which is mediated by the LDL receptor. HDL has diverse origins, its lipid being derived from free cholesterol and phospholipid released during the lipolysis of chylomicrons and VLDL as well as from free cholesterol effluxing from peripheral cells, whereas its major apoprotein, apoA-I, is synthesized both in the liver and small intestine. Nascent HDL particles initially form HDL$_3$ in plasma but eventually get converted to larger HDL$_2$ particles by the action of LCAT, which is activated by apoA-I. Adapted by permission from Thompson, *Br Heart J* 1984, 51:585–588.

2

5.   GOTTO AM, POWNALL HJ, HAVEL RJ: Introduction to the plasma lipoproteins. In *Methods in Enzymology* edited by Segrest JP, Albers JJ. London: Academic Press, 1986, pp 3–41.
A recent, fairly detailed review of all aspects of lipoprotein metabolism.

6.   PACKARD CJ, MUNRO A, LORIMER AR, GOTTO AM, SHEPHERD J: Metabolism of apolipoprotein B in large triglyceride-rich very low density lipoproteins of normal and hypertriglyceridemic subjects. *J Clin Invest* 1984, 74:2178–2192.
Turnover studies which show that the eventual fate of apoB in the circulation is dependent upon the size of the VLDL particle injected.

7.   TENG B, THOMPSON GR, SNIDERMAN AD, FORTE TM, KRAUSS RM, KWITEROVICH PO: Composition and distribution of low density lipoprotein fractions in hyperapobetalipoproteinemia, normolipidemia and familial hypercholesterolemia. *Proc Natl Acad Sci USA* 1983, 80:6662-6666.
Description of a discontinuous density gradient ultracentrifugation method for separating LDL into light and heavy subfractions.

8.   EISENBERG S, LEVY RI: Lipoprotein metabolism. In *Advances in Lipid Research* Vol. 13 edited by Paoletti R, Kritchevsky D. New York: Academic Press, 1975, pp 1–89.
A review of data which enabled the authors to propose the important concept that the partial catabolism of one VLDL particle results in the formation of one LDL particle.

9.   SOUTAR AK, MYANT NB, THOMPSON GR: Simultaneous measurement of apolipoprotein B turnover in very low and low density lipoproteins in familial hypercholesterolaemia. *Atherosclerosis* 1977, 28:247–256.
The first description of direct synthesis of LDL in FH, showing that LDL-apoB synthesis rates were twice as high as VLDL synthesis rates in homozygotes.

10.   HAMILTON RL, WILLIAMS MC, FIELDING CJ, HAVEL RJ: Discoidal bilayer structure of nascent high density lipoproteins from perfused rat liver. *J Clin Invest* 1976, 58:667–680.
Electron micrographic studies of lipoproteins emanating from the perfused rat liver showing that nascent HDL particles are bilayered discs which, by virtue of the action of LCAT, are subsequently converted to spherical, mature HDL_2 particles.

11.   MORRISETT JD, GUYTON TR, GAUBATZ JW, GOTTO AM: Lipoprotein (a): structure, metabolism and epidemiology. In *Plasma Lipoproteins* edited by Gotto AM. Amsterdam: Elsevier Science Publishers, 1987, pp 129–152.
A comprehensive review of a hitherto neglected entity, the importance of which is becoming increasingly apparent.

12.   ENHOLM C, KUUSI T: Preparation, characterization and measurement of hepatic lipase. In *Methods in Enzymology* Vol 129 edited by Albers JJ, Segrest JP. London: Academic Press, 1986, pp 716–738.
An up-to-date review of hepatic lipase.

13.   MCLEAN LR, DEMEE RA, SOCORRO L, SHINOMIYA M, JACKSON RL: Mechanism of action of lipoprotein lipase. In *Methods in Enzymology* Vol 129 edited by Albers JJ, Segrest JP. London: Academic Press, 1986, pp 738–763.
A similarly up-to-date review of extrahepatic lipoprotein lipase.

14.   GLOMSET JA: **Plasma lecithin : cholesterol acyltransferase.** In *Blood Lipids and Lipo-proteins: Quantitation, Composition and Metabolism* edited by Nelson GJ. New York: Wiley Interscience, 1972, pp 745–787.
A classic article which describes the role of LCAT in the so-called Glomset hypothesis of reverse cholesterol transport.

15.   ALBERS JJ, CHEN C-H, LACKO AG: **Isolation, characterization and assay of lecithin-cholesterol acyltransferase.** In *Methods in Enzymology* Vol 129 edited by Albers JJ, Segrest JP. London: Academic Press, 1986, pp 763–783.
A detailed description of the latest findings on the structure of LCAT and the current methods available for isolating and quantifying this important enzyme.

16.   GOLDSTEIN JL, BROWN MS, ANDERSON RGW, RUSSELL DW, SCHNEIDER WJ: **Receptor-mediated endocytosis: concepts emerging from the LDL receptor system.** *Annu Rev Cell Biol* 1985, 1:1–39.
A classic review of the Nobel Prize-winning work on the LDL receptor performed in Dallas over the previous 12 years.

17.   GOLDSTEIN JL, BROWN MS: **Regulation of low density lipoprotein receptors: implications for pathogenesis and therapy of hypercholesterolemia and atherosclerosis.** *Circulation* 1987, 76:504-507.
An abbreviated account of the structure and function of the LDL receptor and its role in health and disease.

18.   BEISIEGEL U, WEBER W, HAVINGA JR, IHRKE G, HUI DY, WERNETTE-HAMMOND ME, TURCK CW, INNERARITY TL, MAHLEY RW: **Apolipoprotein E-binding proteins isolated from dog and human liver.** *Arteriosclerosis* 1988, 8:288–297.
An honest appraisal of data supporting the existence of a chylomicron remnant receptor in the liver but which cannot attribute this role to any of the three apoE-binding proteins discovered so far.

19.   ORAM JF, BRINTON EA, BIERMAN EL: **Regulation of high density lipoprotein receptor activity in cultured human skin fibroblasts and human arterial smooth muscle cells.** *J Clin Invest* 1983, 72:1611–1621.
Description of an HDL receptor in cultured cells which is up regulated by cholesterol loading, in contrast to the classic LDL receptor, and which is proposed to play a major role in reverse cholesterol transport.

20.   HOEG JM, DEMOSKY SJ, EDGE SB, GREGG RE, OSBORNE JC, BREWER HB: **Characterization of a human hepatic receptor for high density lipoproteins.** *Arteriosclerosis* 1985, 5:228–237.
Identification of an HDL-binding receptor in human liver with properties similar to those of the HDL-receptor described in [19].

21.   TOLLEFSON JH, ALBERS JJ: **Isolation, characterization and assay of plasma lipid transfer proteins.** In *Methods in Enzymology* Vol 129 edited by Albers JJ, Segrest JP. London: Academic Press, 1986, pp 797–816.
A useful account of current knowledge about cholesterol ester, triglyceride and phospholipid transfer proteins and how to quantify their activity in human plasma.

2

3 QUANTITATION OF BLOOD LIPIDS AND LIPOPROTEINS

3

Introduction

This chapter describes the methods and general approach used to quantitate the lipid and protein constituents of lipoproteins in plasma rather than the strategy of screening for hyperlipidaemia, which is dealt with in the final chapter.

Lipid analysis

3

Some laboratories prefer to assay lipids in plasma, obtained by addition of EDTA 1 mg/ml to blood to prevent coagulation and subsequent centrifugation, whereas others prefer serum samples. The advantages of using plasma are that EDTA enhances stability of lipoproteins during storage and that the buffy coat of white cells can be kept for subsequent DNA analysis.

Appearance of sample

Values of lipids assayed in serum are approximately 3% higher than those in plasma. Samples can be kept at 4°C for up to 4 days prior to lipid analysis or alternatively can be frozen at −20°C (or preferably −70°C).

The appearance of the plasma or serum will often provide a rough guide to the concentration of triglycerides and whether chylomicrons are present. If the sample is translucent the triglyceride concentration is usually normal (<2.25 mmol/l); if it is hazy the concentration is moderately raised and if opaque or lactescent the value is usually above 6 mmol/l [1]. Chylomicrons form a surface film or layer if the sample is allowed to stand at 4°C; their presence often means that the patient has not fasted. Hypercholesterolaemic samples are translucent but may have an orange colour due to the increase in carotene associated with raised LDL levels.

Cholesterol

Cholesterol can be assayed in whole plasma (or serum) and lipoprotein fractions by either chemical or enzymatic methods. In general, enzymatic procedures have replaced chemical methods of analysis, although the latter are still regarded as the 'gold standard' and are used to assay reference sera. For example, the Centers for Disease Control (CDC) in Atlanta, Georgia use the Abell–Kendall method, which involves solvent extraction of lipids, alkaline hydrolysis of esterified cholesterol and quantitation of total cholesterol by the Lieberman–Burchard reaction, the coloured end product of which is measured spectrophotometrically.

Enzymatic methods involve the conversion of cholesterol esters to free cholesterol and fatty acid by cholesterol esterase and oxidative conversion of free cholesterol to cholesterol-4-ene-3-one and hydrogen peroxide by cholesterol oxidase. The hydrogen peroxide formed is then quantified by various means, which include reaction with phenol and 4-aminophenazone in the presence of peroxidase to form an O-quinoneimine, which can be measured photometrically. These methods are eminently suitable for automation, although the results are reported to be 2.6–4.9% higher than those obtained with the Abell–Kendall reference method [2]. This bias between methods can be corrected by appropriate calibration.

The advent of so-called 'dry chemistry' methodology has led to the development of small portable analysers such as the Reflotron (Boehringer–Mannheim). This machine provides within minutes an estimate of the concentration of cholesterol in a finger-prick sample of capillary blood, and thus has considerable potential in screening for hypercholesterolaemia. Initially the results showed a marked negative bias compared with conventional laboratory methods but subsequent re-calibration of the instrument resulted in an acceptable degree of accuracy being achieved [3]. Other instruments which use a similar approach are the Ektachem DT 60 and the Seralyzer [4].

3

Triglyceride
As with cholesterol so also are there both chemical and enzymatic methods available for triglyceride assay. Chemical methods are tedious because they involve both solvent extraction and removal of phospholipids with solid adsorbents prior to measuring the glycerol released during saponification of triglyceride. Enzymatic methods are far more convenient, albeit also fairly complex in that they involve at least four separate reactions: (1) conversion of triglyceride to glycerol and free fatty acid by lipase; (2) conversion of glycerol and ATP to glycerol-3-phosphate and ADP by glycerol kinase; (3) oxidative conversion of glycerol-3-phosphate to di-hydroxyacetone phosphate and hydrogen peroxide by glycerol phosphate oxidase; (4) conversion of the hydrogen peroxide released during (3) to quinoneimine using peroxidase and photometric quantitation, as in the enzymatic assay of cholesterol [1]. In common with the latter enzymatic assay of triglyceride is easily automated and can also be undertaken with desk-top instruments such as the Reflotron [4].

Caution has to be exercised when assaying triglycerides in two respects. Firstly, blood should not be stored in tubes having glycerol-lubricated stoppers. Secondly, spurious results can occur if higher than normal concentrations of free glycerol happen to be present in the samples to be analysed or in control sera [5].

Criteria of assay performance
The two main criteria of assay performance are accuracy, which is the extent to which the results are biased from the true value, and precision, which is the extent to which an estimate is duplicated upon repeat measurement. Commonly precision is expressed as the coefficient of variation between and within assays, calculated as the standard deviation of repeated measurements divided by their mean.

3

In the LRC Prevalence Study, cholesterol and triglyceride were assayed with the Autoanalyzer II, using chemical methods, and coefficients of variation of <3 and 4%, respectively, were achieved in long-term performance over 10 years [1]. Similarly good precision has recently been reported using automated enzymatic assays [5]. Reference values for serum lipids in white American males and females of various ages obtained during the LRC Prevalence Study are shown in Tables 3.1 and 3.2. Accuracy of these values was assured and monitored using CDC calibration material and rigid performance criteria.

Table 3.1. Plasma lipid and lipoprotein levels in American white males (mmol/l).

Age (years)	Total cholesterol		Triglyceride	
	Mean	5th–95th%	Mean	5th–95th
<10	4.0	3.2–4.9	0.6	0.3–1.0
10–19	4.0	3.1–5.2	0.8	0.4–1.5
20–29	4.5	3.2–5.9	1.1	0.5–2.1
30–39	5.0	3.7–6.8	1.5	0.6–3.2
40–49	5.4	4.0–7.0	1.7	0.6–3.5
50–59	5.6	4.1–7.2	1.6	0.7–3.3
60–69	5.7	4.3–7.5	1.5	0.6–2.9
70+	5.4	3.7–7.0	1.5	0.7–2.9
	LDL cholesterol		HDL cholesterol	
	Mean	5th–95th%	Mean	5th–95th%
<10	1.7	1.7–3.5	1.3	1.0–1.9
10–19	2.5	1.7–3.4	1.3	1.0–1.9
20–29	2.8	1.8–4.3	1.2	0.8–1.7
30–39	3.4	2.1–4.9	1.2	0.8–1.7
40–49	3.6	2.3–5.0	1.2	0.8–1.7
50–59	3.7	2.3–5.2	1.2	0.8–1.7
60–69	3.9	2.5–5.4	1.3	0.8–2.1
70+	3.7	2.3–5.0	1.3	0.8–2.1

Data from Lipid Research Clinics Program (*Circulation* 1979, 60:427–439) and Heiss *et al.* (*Circulation* 1980, 61:302–315).

Recent recommendations emanating from the US National Cholesterol Education Campaign are that, using current methods, inaccuracy should not exceed ±5% and coefficients of variation should be <5%. The need to use reliable sources of reference materials was stressed, as was the desirability of assessing further the performance of desk-top analysers before accepting them as a valid means of screening for hyperlipidaemia [6].

Table 3.2. Plasma lipid and lipoprotein levels in American white females (mmol/l).

Age (years)	Total cholesterol		Triglyceride	
	Mean	5th–95th%	Mean	5th–95th
< 10	4.3	3.4–5.09	1.4	0.8–1.9
10–19	4.1	3.1–5.4	0.8	0.3–1.5
20–29	4.5	3.4–5.9	1.0	0.5–1.9
30–39	4.8	3.5–6.2	1.0	0.5–2.1
40–49	5.2	3.7–6.8	1.2	0.5–2.3
50–59	5.8	4.3–7.5	1.4	0.6–2.9
60–69	6.1	4.4–7.8	1.5	0.6–3.0
70 +	5.8	4.5–7.2	1.5	0.7–3.7
	LDL cholesterol		HDL cholesterol	
	Mean	5th–95th%	Mean	5th–95th%
< 10	2.6	1.8–3.6	1.4	0.8–1.9
10–19	2.5	1.7–3.6	1.3	0.9–1.9
20–29	2.8	1.7–4.3	1.4	0.9–2.1
30–39	3.0	1.8–4.3	1.4	0.9–2.1
40–49	3.2	1.9–4.7	1.6	0.9–2.3
50–59	3.6	2.3–5.4	1.6	0.9–2.5
60–69	3.9	2.5–5.8	1.7	0.9–2.5
70 +	3.9	2.5–5.3	1.6	0.9–2.5

Data from Lipid Research Clinics Program (*Circulation* 1979, 60:427–439) and Heiss *et al.* (*Circulation* 1980, 61:302–315).

3

Separation and determination of lipoproteins

Introduction

Lipoprotein concentrations in plasma or serum are usually expressed in terms of their cholesterol content, determined after preliminary isolation by ultracentrifugation or precipitation or a combination of both. Additional qualitative information can sometimes be obtained by lipoprotein electrophoresis. All three approaches were used in the LRC Program, as described in detail elsewhere [7]. However, in routine clinical practice there is an increasing tendency nowadays to dispense with ultracentrifugation and instead to derive values for VLDL and LDL cholesterol by applying the formula of Friedewald *et al.* [8]. This formula is based on two assumptions: (1) that most of the triglyceride in plasma is located in VLDL; (2) that the mass ratio of triglyceride:cholesterol in VLDL is 5:1 (molar ratio 2.19:1) except in type III hyperlipoproteinaemia or in the presence of marked hypertriglyceridaemia (> 4.5 mmol/l), when the formula is known to be inaccurate. However, apart from these exceptions it provides a reasonably accurate means of calculating LDL cholesterol, as follows:

$$\text{LDL cholesterol} = \text{total cholesterol} - \text{HDL cholesterol} - \frac{\text{triglyceride}}{2.2} \text{ mmol/l}$$

The increasing tendency to use calculated LDL cholesterol values when assessing risk underlines the importance of high degrees of accuracy and precision in relation to laboratory measurement of total and HDL cholesterol, and triglyceride [6]. It should also be obvious that LDL cholesterol will be underestimated if a non-fasting triglyceride value is used in the Friedewald formula.

Ultracentrifugation

Preparative ultracentrifugation is routinely used to isolate lipoproteins for research purposes and is also used in the differential diagnosis of the severe or unusual hyperlipidaemias occasionally seen in a clinical setting. Analytical ultracentrifugation of lipoproteins is purely used for research purposes and is undertaken by only a handful of laboratories throughout the world, as is zonal ultracentrifugation. Recent reviews of both procedures have been published elsewhere [9,10].

Isolation of lipoproteins by preparative ultracentrifugation commonly involves their sequential flotation after adjustment of the background density of plasma or serum by addition of sodium chloride (d 1.006) alone or mixed with a potassium bromide/sodium chloride solution (d 1.346), as first described by Havel *et al.* [11]. Thus VLDL can be isolated at d 1.006, IDL at d 1.019, LDL at d 1.063 and HDL at d 1.21. Depending upon the centrifugal force applied (which depends upon the type of rotor and speed of centrifugation), each separation takes between 12 and 36 hours in most angled head rotors at 10°C. At the end of each spin the supernatant lipoprotein fraction is separated from the infranatant by tube slicing, using a special knife, or by aspiration with a pipette. The harvested lipoproteins are then made up to a convenient volume and assayed for their lipid and protein content, as required, or subjected to lipoprotein electrophoresis. There are also small, air-driven ultracentrifuges which now enable separation of lipoproteins in less than 6 hours.

In the LRC Program [7] plasma was routinely centrifuged at its own background density of 1.006. The cholesterol content of the LDL plus HDL (d > 1.006) was then measured and subtracted from plasma total cholesterol to obtain VLDL cholesterol. HDL cholesterol was determined separately, by a precipitation method, and subtraction of its value from d > 1.006 cholesterol gave the value of LDL cholesterol. Direct measurement of d < 1.006 cholesterol was regarded as too inaccurate to be used as a measure of VLDL cholesterol but the ratio of cholesterol : triglyceride and electrophoretic mobility of the d < 1.006 fraction are useful in the diagnosis of type III hyperlipoproteinaemia.

Discontinuous density gradient ultracentrifugation provides a means of separating all the major lipoprotein fractions in a single spin in a swinging bucket rotor and involves the creation of a step-wise gradient by manual addition of solutions of differing density [12]. It can also be used to isolate LDL subfractions (Fig. 3.1).

3

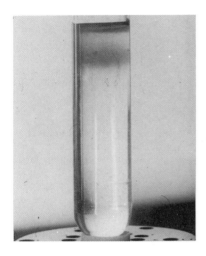

Fig. 3.1. Light (upper) and heavy (lower) subfractions of LDL after discontinuous density gradient ultracentrifugation for 40 hours at 10°C in a Beckman SW 50.1 rotor.

A recent innovation which greatly reduces the time taken to separate lipoproteins in the ultracentrifuge is the technique of vertical spin density gradient ultracentrifugation [13]. This involves first increasing the density of plasma by the addition of solid potassium bromide, using a formula based on the partial specific volume of that salt [14], and overlayering the mixture with less dense sodium chloride. The two-step gradient is then centrifuged in a vertical rotor in an ultracentrifuge fitted with a slow start and stop mechanism. Depending upon the size of rotor used it takes between 40 min and $2\frac{1}{2}$ hours to isolate LDL. This is also a useful means of isolating Lp(a), which has a density intermediate between LDL and HDL, as illustrated in Fig. 3.2.

Precipitation

The use of polyanion-divalent cation mixtures to precipitate lipoproteins has been described in detail by Burstein and Scholnick [15]. For present purposes discussion of this approach will be limited to its use in the measurement of cholesterol in HDL and its subfractions.

Quantitation of HDL cholesterol depends upon initial precipitation of VLDL and LDL followed by analysis of cholesterol in the HDL-containing supernatant. The ideal method is one which completely precipitates all lipoproteins except HDL. No such method exists in that they all precipitate the apoE-rich

3

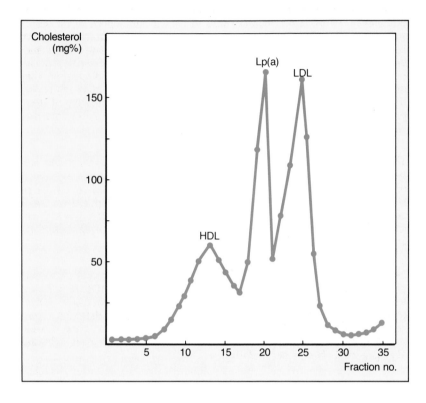

Fig. 3.2. Distribution of cholesterol in the fractions obtained after centrifugation of Lp(a) containing plasma in a vertical rotor at 65 000 r.p.m. for 1½ hours. Adapted by permission [13].

fraction of HDL (HDL₁), whereas this is recovered along with the remainder of HDL if HDL cholesterol is measured in the d 1.063–1.21 fraction of plasma. However, ultracentrifugation can give spuriously high values for HDL cholesterol in samples containing much Lp(a) whereas the latter is removed by precipitation procedures.

In the original LRC method 200 i.u. of heparin was added to each ml of plasma plus sufficient MnCl₂ to give a final concentration of 46 mM [7]. After standing for 30 min in ice the mixture was centrifuged at 1500 **g** for 30 min at 4°C and the supernatant pipetted off for analysis of the cholesterol content of a measured aliquot, the value being corrected to allow for the dilution of each ml of sample by 0.1 ml of reagents.

More complete precipitation of apoB-containing lipoproteins is achieved by doubling the final concentration of $MnCl_2$ to 92 mM, especially in plasma stored for a few days. Serum analysed by this modified method should have EDTA added first. One drawback of both methods is that manganese sometimes interferes with subsequent enzymatic analysis of cholesterol. This can be overcome by addition of EDTA to the diluent used in analysers. Another drawback is their inability to precipitate VLDL completely in markedly hypertriglyceridaemic samples, which necessitates either having to filter floating precipitates, or diluting or even ultracentrifuging the sample before the precipitation step.

3

These problems can be largely overcome by instead adding dextran sulphate (MW 50 000) and $MgCl_2$ to plasma or serum, in final concentrations of 0.91 mg/ml and 45 mM, respectively [16]. This method gives values of HDL cholesterol which are virtually identical to those obtained with the modified heparin-manganese procedure, and when used in conjunction with automated enzymatic analysis of cholesterol a coefficient of variation of < 4% is achievable [5].

Dual precipitation methods for quantitating HDL subfractions involve first precipitating apoB-containing lipoproteins, which enables HDL total cholesterol to be determined, and then precipitating HDL_2, which enables HDL_3 cholesterol to be measured. HDL_2 is then calculated by difference. Two such methods have been developed, one using heparin-$MnCl_2$ and dextran sulphate, the other using two different concentrations of dextran sulphate-$MgCl_2$, as described in detail elsewhere [16].

Electrophoresis
Lipoprotein electrophoresis in the LRC Program was performed on paper but nowadays agarose gel is the preferred support medium, as originally described by Noble [17]. This involves mixing 8.2 ml of a 1% solution of agarose in barbitone buffer with 5.7 ml buffer and 0.3 ml 30% bovine serum albumin at 60°C. The gel is then spread on to a glass plate and allowed to dry. Samples of serum are applied to the gel and electrophoresed for $2\frac{1}{4}$ hours. The plate is then fixed and stained with Sudan Black. If chylomicrons are present they remain at the origin but in fasting samples the three main bands in order of increasing mobility represent LDL (β), VLDL (preβ) and HDL (α). A significant amount of Lp(a) in plasma or in the d > 1.006 ultracentrifugal fraction gives rise to a band between LDL and VLDL (preβ_1 or 'sinking' preβ lipoprotein). The presence of a band with β-mobility in the d < 1.006 fraction ('floating' β) is pathognomonic of type III hyperlipoproteinaemia, which is also characterized by the presence of a broad β-band in serum (Fig. 3.3). Attempts to quantitate lipoproteins after electrophoresis by densitometry are not recommended and nowadays the procedure is used mainly to help differentiate between type III and other types of severe hypertriglyceridaemia.

3

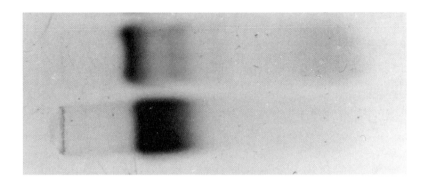

Fig. 3.3 Agarose gel electrophoresis of fasting plasma from a normal subject (upper) and a type III patient (lower). The latter characteristically shows the presence of chylomicrons at the origin (left), a broad β-band and virtual absence of α-lipoprotein (HDL). Published by permission of Dr Iris Trayner.

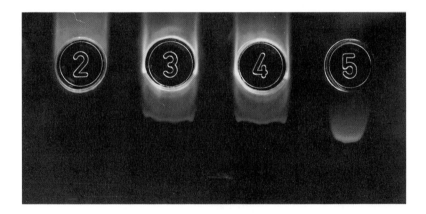

Fig. 3.4. Agar gel electrophoresis of normal plasma (2), LCAT deficient plasma (3 and 4) and plasma from a patient with primary biliary cirrhosis (5). Lipoprotein-X is seen migrating towards the cathode (downwards) in wells 3, 4 and 5. Published by permission of Dr Iris Trayner.

One other instance where lipoprotein electrophoresis is useful is in diagnosing the presence of lipoprotein X, an abnormal lipoprotein found in patients with biliary obstruction and also in familial LCAT deficiency. Lipoprotein X differs from all other lipoproteins in that it migrates in the opposite direction, i.e. cathodally, on agar gel (Fig. 3.4).

Apolipoprotein assays

Introduction

Measurement of apolipoproteins as indices of coronary heart disease (CHD) risk, especially apoA-I and apoB, is rapidly gaining in popularity. This approach is rational in that the concentration of individual apoproteins provides a better index of the number of particles present in plasma than does measurement of lipoprotein cholesterol, which is influenced by changes in lipoprotein composition as well as in concentration. However, most of the existing epidemiological data relating risk of CHD to lipoprotein levels are based on lipid measurements; almost no prospective data are available to evaluate apolipoproteins as predictors of CHD. Other drawbacks to the widespread adoption of apolipoprotein measurements are the multiplicity of methods available, the variability of results between different laboratories and the difficulty in standardization of assays, for reasons discussed elsewhere [1]. Nevertheless when these problems are sorted out it is likely that apolipoprotein quantitation will become an integral part of the assessment of CHD risk, not least because of the ease and speed with which the relevant immunochemical assays can be performed on large numbers of samples.

ApoA-I, apoB and Lp(a)

At present the main focus of interest is in developing valid methods of assaying apoB, apoA-I and Lp(a). The pros and cons of the various methods available for this purpose are discussed below but all are subject to limitations imposed by the structure of the lipoproteins themselves. One drawback is that the antigenic expression of apoB in VLDL is much less than in LDL unless the VLDL is first subjected to partial lipolysis or unless monoclonal antibodies to epitopes of apoB fully expressed in both VLDL and LDL are used. To a lesser extent a similar problem besets apoA-I in HDL, although this can be largely overcome by partially delipidating HDL with tetramethylurea (TMU) or Tween 20. Lp(a) contains two apoproteins and although it is possible to measure apo(a) using antisera from which all anti-apoB activity has been adsorbed, nevertheless the apoB in Lp(a) will be measured together with that in LDL when assaying apoB in plasma. A detailed consideration of such problems and the development of a potential reference and calibration material has recently been undertaken by the Lipid-Apoprotein Subcommittee of the International Union of Immunological Societies [18–20].

Radio-immunoassay

This method has the advantage that it uses minimal amounts of antisera, can utilize monoclonal antibodies or polyvalent antisera, and is extremely sensitive. Its disadvantages are that its sensitivity necessitates large sample dilutions, it is potentially hazardous in that it uses radiation (usually ^{125}I), requires continual upkeep because of reagent instability, and offers only moderate precision. However, radio-immunoassay remains the potential reference procedure for apolipoprotein measurements and is extremely useful for measurements of apolipoproteins which occur in much lower concentrations in plasma than apoA-I and B.

Radial immunodiffusion

The advantages of radial immunodiffusion (RID) are that it is technically simple and requires inexpensive equipment. It has fairly good precision and requires small sample dilutions. It does, however, have significant disadvantages for apolipoprotein measurements in requiring a specific antibody which can achieve good precipitation, usually achievable only with polyvalent antisera, and in using large amounts of antiserum. There is variable migration of different lipoproteins through the support media, depending on particle size, and this may necessitate sample manipulation prior to analysis. It is also a slow and rather tedious procedure. Although RID is probably not an optimal method for apoA-I, it is useful for measuring apoB in LDL, but not in VLDL, as shown in Fig. 3.5. It has also been used to assay Lp(a) [21].

Immunonephelometric assays

There are significant advantages to immunonephelometric assays in the clinical laboratory in that the procedure is extremely rapid and can handle large sample numbers. It is easily automated and the cost per assay is relatively low. The precision is generally good and the assay systems require minimal upkeep. The disadvantages relate to the intrinsic limitations of a technique that depends on measurement of light scattering, whether measuring rate or endpoint, because samples with elevated lipoprotein concentrations are themselves inherently light scattering. Polyvalent antisera are usually needed to achieve precipitation or at least lattice formation and as the technique is sensitive, large sample dilutions are required. However, these procedures have become extremely popular due to the fact that they are rapid, provide large sample throughput and can easily be automated [22].

Electroimmunoassay

The advantages of electroimmunoassay (EIA) or rocket immunoelectrophoresis are that it requires minimal upkeep, samples need only be diluted 10–40-fold and the equipment is relatively inexpensive. There are, however, significant disadvantages which include the slowness of the procedures, the limited number of assays that can be performed in a given period, the need for large amounts of precipitating polyvalent antisera, and only moderate precision.

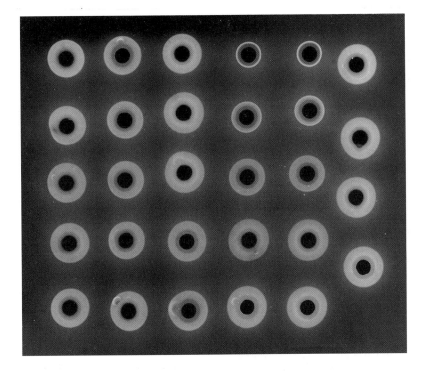

3

Fig. 3.5. Radial immunodiffusion assay of apoB, showing variation in diameter of rings around each well according to the concentration of apoB added. Stained with 1% tannic acid. By courtesy of Dr Iris Trayner.

Enzyme-linked immunosorbent assay

The potential advantages of enzyme-linked immunosorbent assays (ELISAs) are considerable. They are highly automatable and offer a sensitivity close to that of radio-immunoassay but require minimal upkeep as the reagents are extremely stable. The assays are rapid, allowing high throughput. They can be developed with both monoclonal antibodies [23] and polyvalent antisera. ELISA procedures can utilize either a competitive system or a capture (sandwich) assay. They require minimal amounts of antibody and, when automated, have good precision. The disadvantages are that for automation, expensive and relatively unique equipment is required and the antibody used in detection, either in a competitive or a capture assay, requires labelling. Large sample dilutions similar to that for radio-immunoassay may be required, especially in the capture assays. However, dilutions on a more modest scale (200–400-fold) can be utilized in the competitive systems.

Annotated references

3

1.   STEIN EA: **Lipids, lipoproteins and apolipoproteins.** In *Textbook of Clinical Chemistry* edited by Tietz NW. Philadelphia: W.B. Saunders, 1986, pp 829–900.
A detailed description of the methods used to measure plasma lipid and lipoprotein concentrations in the clinical chemistry laboratory.

2.   KROLL MH, LINDSEY H, GREENE J, SILVA C, HAINLINE A, ELIN RJ: **Bias between enzymatic methods and the reference method for cholesterol.** *Clin Chem* 1988, 34:131–135.
Comparison in over 300 samples of the Abell–Kendall method with four enzymatic methods of measuring cholesterol showed a positive bias in three of them.

3.   BOERMA GJM, VAN GORP I, LIEM TL, LEIJNSE B, BEUM J, CARSTENSEN CA: **Revised calibration of the Reflotron cholesterol assay evaluated.** *Clin Chem* 1988, 34:1124–1127.
An appraisal of the re-calibrated Reflotron system shows it to have acceptable levels of accuracy and precision.

4.   VON SCHENCK H, TREICHL L, TILLING B, OLSSON AG: **Laboratory and field evaluation of three desk-top instruments for assay of cholesterol and triglyceride.** *Clin Chem* 1987, 33:1230–1232.
Evaluation of the Ektachem DT 60, Reflotron and Seralyzer 'dry chemistry' instruments available for lipid analysis.

5.   MCNAMARA JR, SCHAEFER EJ: **Automated enzymatic standardized lipid analyses for plasma and lipoprotein fractions.** *Clin Chim Acta* 1987, 166:1–8.
Impressive standards of accuracy and precision were achieved by the authors using automated enzymatic analysis of cholesterol and triglyceride combined with dextran sulphate-magnesium chloride precipitation for measurement of HDL cholesterol.

6.   **Current status of blood cholesterol measurement in clinical laboratories in the United States: a report from the Laboratory Standardization Panel of the National Cholesterol Education Program.** *Clin Chem* 1988, 34:193–201.
Important recommendations regarding acceptable levels of accuracy and precision in measuring serum lipids in clinical laboratories in the USA at present and proposals for the future.

7.   *Manual of Laboratory Operations, Lipid Research Clinics Program. Vol I: Lipid and Lipoprotein Analysis.* DHEW Publication 1974, No (NIH) 75–628.
Rapidly becoming a historic document, this manual provides a detailed account of the methods used by the LRC during the 1970s.

8.   FRIEDEWALD WT, LEVY RI, FREDRICKSON DS: **Estimation of the concentration of low-density lipoprotein cholesterol in plasma, without use of the preparative ultracentrifuge.** *Clin Chem* 1972, 18:499–502.
The Friedewald formula was based upon analysis of 450 samples, correlation between calculated and ultracentrifugally isolated LDL cholesterol values being best with normal and hypercholesterolaemic plasma, less good with hypertriglyceridaemic samples.

9.   KAHLON TS, GLINES LA, LINDGREN FT: **Analytic ultracentrifugation of plasma lipo-proteins.** In *Methods in Enzymology* edited by Albers JJ, Segrest JP. London: Academic Press 1986, **129**:26–45.
A description of analytical ultracentrifugation by one of the pioneers of this technique, Frank Lindgren, and colleagues from the Donner Laboratory.

10.   PATSCH JR, PATSCH W: **Zonal ultracentrifugation.** In *Methods in Enzymology* edited by Albers JJ, Segrest JP. London: Academic Press 1986, **129**:3–21.
A description of zonal ultracentrifugation as exploited by the Patsch brothers to study lipo-protein metabolism.

11.   HAVEL RJ, EDER HA, BRAGDON JH: **The distribution and chemical composition of ultracentrifugally separated lipoproteins in human serum.** *J Clin Invest* 1955, **34**:1345–1353.
A classic paper describing the use of preparative ultracentrifugation to separate the major classes of lipoproteins found in human and animal plasma.

12.   KELLEY JL, KRUSKI AW: **Density gradient ultracentrifugation of serum lipoproteins in a swinging bucket rotor.** In *Methods in Enzymology* edited by Segrest JP, Albers JJ. London: Academic Press 1986, **126**:170–181.
Description of a technique which enables separation of all the major lipoprotein classes and subspecies thereof in a single ultracentrifugal spin.

13.   CHUNG BH, SEGREST JP, RAY MJ, BRUNZELL JD, HOKANSON JE, KRAUSS RM, BEAUDRIE K, CONE JT: **Single vertical spin density gradient ultracentrifugation.** In *Methods in Enzymology* edited by Segrest JP, Albers JJ. London: Academic Press 1986, **128**:181–209.
The invention of the vertical rotor has greatly shortened the duration of ultracentrifugation required to separate LDL from HDL.

14.   HATCH FT, LEES RS: **Practical methods for plasma lipoprotein analysis.** *Adv Lipid Res* 1968, **6**:1–68.
A review of methods used to study lipoproteins 20 years ago, some of which are still useful.

15.   BURSTEIN M, SCHOLNICK HR: **Lipoprotein-polyanion-metal interactions.** *Adv Lipid Res* 1973, **11**:67–108.
Description of the use of polyanions and divalent cations to precipitate not only VLDL and LDL but also HDL, as first developed by Burstein.

16.   BACHORIK PS, ALBERS JJ: **Precipitation methods for quantification of lipoproteins.** In *Methods in Enzymology* edited by Albers JJ, Segrest JP. London: Academic Press 1986, **129**:78–100.
Useful appraisal of acceptable methods for measuring HDL cholesterol and its subfractions after first precipitating VLDL and LDL.

17.   NOBLE RP: **Electrophoretic separation of plasma lipoproteins in agarose gel.** *J Lipid Res* 1968, **9**:693–700.
First description of the use of agarose gel electrophoresis to separate lipoproteins.

3

18.   STEINBERG KK, COOPER GR, GRAISER SR, ROSSENEU M: Some considerations of methodology and standardization of apolipoprotein A-I immunoassays. *Clin Chem* 1983, 29:415–426.
See [20].

19.   ROSSENEU M, VERCAEMST R, STEINBERG KK, COOPER GR: Some considerations of methodology and standardization of apolipoprotein B immunoassays. *Clin Chem* 1983, 29:427–433.
See [20].

20.   SMITH SJ, COOPER GR, HENDERSON LO, HANNON WH AND THE APOLIPOPROTEIN STANDARDIZATION COLLABORATING GROUP: An international collaborative study on standardization of apolipoproteins A-I and B. Part 1. Evaluation of a lyophilized candidate reference and calibration material. *Clin Chem* 1987, 33:2240–2249.
These three papers examine in considerable detail the various methods available for quantitating apoA-I and apoB and describe the development of a reference material for use in the standardization of such assays.

21.   ALBERS JJ, HAZZARD WR: Immunochemical quantification of human plasma Lp(a). *Lipids* 1974, 9:15–26.
Measurement of Lp(a) in plasma using an RID assay.

22.   MACIEJKO JJ, LEVINSON SS, MARKYVECH L, SMITH MP, BLEVINS RD: New assay of apolipoproteins A-I and B by rate nephelometry evaluated. *Clin Chem* 1987, 33:2065–2069.
An evaluation of the Beckman ICS Analyzer II which performs rate immunonephelometric quantitation of apoA-I and apoB with reasonable precision and accuracy.

23.   YOUNG SG, SMITH RD, HOGLE DM, CURTISS LK, WITZTUM JL: Two new monoclonal antibody-based enzyme-linked assays of apolipoprotein B. *Clin Chem* 1986, 32:1484–1490.
Monoclonal antibody-based one-step direct and two-step competitive ELISAs for apoB, not requiring isotopic labelling.

4 LIPOPROTEIN AND APOLIPOPROTEIN PHENOTYPES

4

Classification of hyperlipidaemia

Introduction
The emergence of lipidology on the clinical scene can be said to have occurred in 1967 when Fredrickson, Levy and Lees [1] introduced their classification of hyperlipidaemia. Prior to that there had been no real appreciation
that hypercholesterolaemia and hypertriglyceridaemia simply reflected alterations in lipoprotein metabolism and previous workers had focused their
attention mainly on the biochemistry of the lipids involved. One exception
to this rule was Gofman who, with his colleagues at the Donner Laboratory,
used analytical ultracentrifugation to quantitate the concentration of lipoproteins of S$_f$ 0–12, 12–20, 20–100 and 100–400 in patients with various forms
of hyperlipidaemia, both primary and secondary [2]. However, analytical ultracentrifugation was far too cumbersome a technique for routine use in the
investigation of hyperlipidaemia. Using much simpler methods, including paper electrophoresis and preparative ultracentrifugation, Fredrickson et al. [1]
described five phenotypic patterns of hyperlipoproteinaemia. Following crit-
icisms that five types were insufficient to encompass all varieties of hyperlip-

idaemia [3] the classification was subsequently revised by the World Health Organization (WHO) to include an additional phenotype [4].

WHO classification

The WHO system provides a convenient shorthand means of describing the lipoprotein profile of most commonly occurring patterns of hyperlipidaemia but does not specify whether the cause is genetically determined or is secondary to environmental factors or underlying disease. It should also be understood that the lipoprotein phenotype of an individual with hyperlipidaemia can change from one pattern to another in response to changes in diet, body weight or treatment. The classification took no account of variations in HDL cholesterol although it subsequently became clear that these have considerable bearing on the likelihood that an individual with hyperlipidaemia will develop CHD, as discussed in the next chapter. Despite these limitations the typing system has had a major influence in directing attention to the nature of the metabolic defects involved in hyperlipidaemia, thus promoting a rational approach to diagnosis and treatment. Attempts by others to simplify the classification of hyperlipidaemia have not met with much success and despite its imperfections the WHO system continues to be widely used by clinicians.

Lipoprotein phenotyping

Criteria

The basic requirements for determining the lipoprotein phenotype are measurement of the levels of triglyceride, total cholesterol and LDL cholesterol in fasting plasma. Alternatively, LDL cholesterol can be calculated (see Chapter 3), after first measuring HDL cholesterol. In addition it is necessary to inspect obviously lipaemic samples to differentiate between chylomicrons and VLDL [3] and to undertake lipoprotein electrophoresis if type III hyperlipoproteinaemia is suspected (see Fig. 3.3).

One of the key determinants of lipoprotein phenotype is whether the LDL cholesterol is or is not raised. Hazzard *et al.* [5] used age-related cut-offs but the current trend is to regard an LDL cholesterol of > 4.1 mmol/l, irrespective of age, as representing a high risk, at least in the USA [6]. The definition of what constitutes abnormality is inevitably arbitrary and a value of LDL cholesterol which is regarded as normal in one country might be considered unacceptably high in another. Most authorities would agree than an LDL cholesterol value of 5 mmol/l or above is definitely associated with increased risk of atherosclerosis and we will therefore use this as our cut-off, together with upper limits for total cholesterol and fasting triglyceride of 6.5 and 2 mmol/l, respectively, when defining phenotypes.

As shown in Table 4.1 the type I phenotype indicates hypertriglyceridaemia due to chylomicronaemia; in type IIa the hypercholesterolaemia is due to an increase in LDL cholesterol whereas in type IIb this increase in LDL cholesterol is accompanied by mild to moderate hypertriglyceridaemia, denoting an increase in VLDL; in type III serum cholesterol and triglyceride are both raised, due to accumulation of chylomicron remnants and IDL; in type IV fasting hypertriglyceridaemia, due to an increase in VLDL, is often accompanied by mild to moderate hypercholesterolaemia but the LDL cholesterol is normal; and in type V marked hypertriglyceridaemia is due both to chylomicronaemia and an increase in VLDL.

4

Table 4.1. World Health Organization classification of hyperlipoproteinaemia.

Type	Plasma cholesterol	LDL cholesterol	Plasma triglyceride	Lipoprotein abnormality
I	Raised	Low or normal	Raised	Excess chylomicrons
IIa	Raised or normal	Raised	Normal	Excess LDL
IIb	Raised	Raised	Raised	Excess LDL and VLDL
III	Raised	Low or normal	Raised	Excess chylomicron remnants and IDL
IV	Raised or normal	Normal	Raised	Excess VLDL
V	Raised	Normal	Raised	Excess chylomicrons and VLDL

Causes

Each of these phenotypes can be either primary or secondary, as shown in Table 4.2. Often, there is interaction between genetic factors and environmental influences, including diet and drugs. Frequently the inherited component is polygenically determined and therefore rather ill-defined but at least three clearly inherited disorders have been described, familial hypercholesterolaemia, familial type III hyperlipoproteinaemia and familial combined hyperlipidaemia, as discussed in subsequent chapters.

Differentiation between the severe hypertriglyceridaemia of types I and V hyperlipoproteinaemia can be achieved by visual inspection, as shown in Fig. 4.1. As mentioned previously lipoprotein electrophoresis is useful in determining whether an individual with moderate or marked elevation of cholesterol and triglyceride has type III hyperlipoproteinaemia. The characteristic broad β band of this phenotype is shown in Fig. 4.2, together with the appearance of all the others except type I.

4

Table 4.2. Aetiology of lipoprotein phenotypes.

Type	Primary causes	Secondary causes
I	Lipoprotein lipase deficiency Apoc-II deficiency	Systemic lupus erythematosus (rare)
IIa IIb	Familial hypercholesterolaemia, Familial combined hyperlipidaemia	Hypothyroidism Nephrotic syndrome Diabetes Anorexia nervosa
III	Familial type III hyperlipoproteinaemia	Hypothyroidism Diabetes, Obesity
IV V	Familial combined hyperlipidaemia, Familial hypertriglyceridaemia Familial hypertriglyceridaemia Apoc-II deficiency	Diabetes Chronic renal disease Alcohol Diuretics, Beta blockers Oral contraceptive

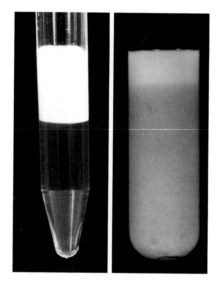

Fig. 4.1. Characteristic appearance on standing in the cold of plasma from type I patient (left) showing chylomicrons and clear subnatant, and from type V patient (right) showing chylomicrons and opalescent infranatant due to increased VLDL.

Unclassified abnormalities

Before concluding the section on lipoprotein phenotyping it is necessary to comment briefly on two matters which are not dealt with in the WHO classification. Firstly, it is important to determine whether an individual with hyperlipidaemia has a reduced level of HDL cholesterol, which carries an increased

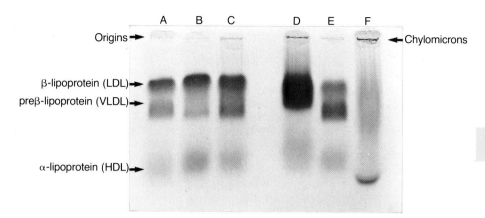

Fig. 4.2. Agarose gel electrophoresis of serum from patients with normal (A), type IIa (B), type IIb (C), type III (D), type IV (E) and type V (F) lipoprotein phenotypes. By courtesy of Dr Iris Trayner. Published by permission from *Clinical Nutrition in Paediatric Disorders* edited by Bentley and Lawson. Baillière Tindall.

risk of CHD, or an increased level, which is harmless or possibly even beneficial. Secondly, it is now apparent that some individuals with a normal LDL cholesterol, especially those with hypertriglyceridaemia, i.e. a type IV phenotype, have an increased concentration of LDL-apoB in their plasma. This apparent paradox is due to the presence of increased numbers of smaller than normal, cholesterol ester-depleted but potentially atherogenic LDL particles and is termed hyperapoβlipoproteinaemia [7]. Thus any evaluation of lipoprotein phenotype ideally should include the results of HDL cholesterol and LDL-apoB measurements. In fact there is a good case for defining an increased HDL cholesterol (> 2 mmol/l) or hyperαlipoproteinaemia as a lipoprotein phenotype in its own right (type VI), differing from all the others in not requiring treatment provided LDL is not elevated.

Apolipoprotein E phenotypes

ApoE polymorphism was first described by Utermann *et al.* [8], using isoelectric focusing of delipidated VLDL. Zannis and Breslow [9] subsequently used two-dimensional electrophoresis and neuraminidase treatment to desialate the sialated forms of apoE, and proposed that the latter was inherited at a single locus with three common alleles. The conflicting terminologies of the two groups of workers were subsequently resolved and resulted in the current, generally accepted classification under which the commonly occurring alleles are termed ε2, 3 and 4 [10].

The frequency of the various alleles varies between populations but in all instances the commonest pattern is homozygosity for ε3, giving rise to an apoE3/3 phenotype (55%), with apoE3/4 as the next most common phenotype (26%). The least frequently occurring phenotype involving these three alleles is apoE2/2 (1%), which in some instance is associated with type III hyperlipoproteinaemia [11]. The appearance of each of the six common phenotypes after isoelectric focusing of delipidated VLDL [12] is shown in Fig. 4.3. Other much rarer isoforms which have also been described are apoE1 and apoE5 [13].

Although originally used as a research tool, apoE phenotyping is rapidly becoming an important diagnostic aid, especially in the diagnosis of type III hyperlipoproteinaemia, and can now be achieved without ultracentrifugation [14]. In addition there is evidence that subjects with the ε4 allele have higher LDL cholesterol levels than those with the normal apoE3/3 pattern [15]. For a detailed description of apoE polymorphism and its genetic basis see [16].

ApoA-I variants

At least seven variants of apoA-I have been identified so far, due to either mutations or deletions of single amino acids [16]. In one instance (apoA-I_{Milano}) this has resulted in decreased HDL cholesterol but the remainder are associated with normal levels. In addition a family has been described in which a large mutation affecting both the apoA-I and CIII gene loci resulted in complete absence of apoA-I and CIII from plasma, very low HDL cholesterol levels and premature CHD. Identification of some apoA-I polymorphisms can be achieved by isoelectric focusing; this has obvious applications in the investigation of hypoαlipoproteinaemia. It remains to be seen whether alterations in apoA-I ever give rise to hyperα-lipoproteinaemia.

Differentiation of apoB$_{100}$ and apoB$_{48}$

The two forms of apoB can be readily separated by means of sodium dodecyl sulphate-polyacrylamide gel electrophoresis, apoB$_{48}$ having greater mobility than apoB$_{100}$. However, it is not easy to determine the relative amounts of

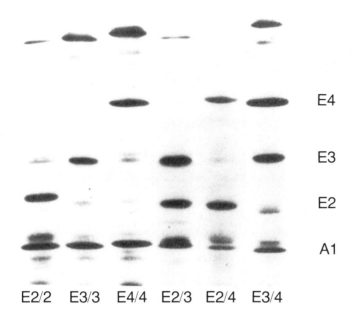

4

E4

E3

E2

A1

E2/2   E3/3   E4/4   E2/3   E2/4   E3/4

Fig. 4.3. The six common apoE phenotypes determined by isoelectric focusing polyacrylamide gel electrophoresis. Published by permission from Gregg and Brewer, *Clin Chem* 1988, 34:B28–B32, B123–B132. © American Association for Clinical Chemistry, Inc.

each because of their differing chromogenicity when stained with Coomassie Blue [17]. Nor is it possible to quantitate apoB$_{48}$ separately from apoB$_{100}$ by immunochemical means, in that the former represents the aminoterminal portion of the latter. Measuring total apoB and then subtracting apoB$_{100}$ using a monoclonal antibody directed against the carboxyterminal portion of apoB$_{100}$ to measure the latter, provides a possible approach but the concentration of apoB$_{48}$ in plasma is so much less than that of apoB$_{100}$ as to render this liable to large errors.

Lp(a) phenotypes

Utermann *et al.* [18] have shown that apo(a) is polymorphic on SDS-PAGE electrophoresis under reducing conditions with immunoblotting. They demonstrated considerable variations in the apparent molecular weight of apo(a) and described six commonly occurring phenotypes, which they designated according to the mobility of apo(a) relative to apoB$_{100}$ (B = same, S1–4 = slower in varying degrees). Of great interest is their observation that

Table 4.3. Apo(a) phenotype frequencies and Lp(a) concentrations (mean ± s.d.) in Austrian blood donors.

Apo(a) phenotype	Frequency	Lp(a) (mg/dl plasma)*
B	1.6%	61.7 ± 7.8
S1	4.2%	23.5 ± 19
S2	14.4%	26.3 ± 21
S3	12.9%	11.3 ± 7.1
S4	21.6%	10.2 ± 6.1
'O'	37.6%	4.4 ± 4.9

*By electroimmunoassay. Published by permission from [18].

4

the concentration of Lp(a) in plasma varies according to the apo(a) phenotype of the individuals concerned, as illustrated in Table 4.3. Those with no detectable band on immunoblotting were designated as having a null ('0') phenotype and had the lowest concentrations of Lp(a) in plasma. The mean concentration varied among the other phenotypes being highest in Lp(a)^B, which has the lowest apparent molecular weight of the six. These findings are especially important in view of the increased risk of CHD associated with high levels of Lp(a), as discussed in the next chapter.

Annotated references

1.   FREDRICKSON DS, LEVY RI, LEES RS: Fat transport in lipoproteins — an integrated approach to mechanisms and disorders. *N Engl J Med* 1967, 276:34–44; 94–103; 148–156; 215–224; 273–281.
A seminal series of five articles which interpreted hyperlipidaemia in terms of underlying changes in lipoprotein metabolism.

2.   GOFMAN JW, RUBIN L, MCGINLEY JP, JONES HB: Hyperlipoproteinemia. *Am J Med* 1954, 17:514–520.
The first demonstration that different forms of hyperlipidaemia were associated with different patterns of lipoprotein abnormality, using analytical ultracentrifugation.

3.   HAVEL RJ: Typing of hyperlipoproteinemias. *Atherosclerosis* 1970, 11:3–6.
An early editorial appraisal of the Fredrickson *et al* classification.

4.   BEAUMONT JL, CARLSON LA, COOPER GR, FEJFAR Z, FREDRICKSON DS, STRASSER T: Classification of hyperlipidaemias and hyperlipoproteinaemias. *Bull WHO* 1970, 43:891–908.
The revised version of the classification of lipoprotein phenotypes which subdivides type II into IIa and IIb.

5. HAZZARD WR, GOLDSTEIN JL, SCHROTT HG, MOTULSKY AG, BIERMAN EL: **Hyperlipidemia in coronary heart disease. III. Evaluation of lipoprotein phenotypes of 156 genetically defined survivors of myocardial infarction.** *J Clin Invest* 1973, 52:1569–1577.
A description of lipoprotein phenotyping in survivors of myocardial infarction and their relatives which concluded that there was no consistent relationship between lipoprotein phenotype and the underlying genetic disorder.

6. EXPERT PANEL: **Report of the National Cholesterol Education Program Expert Panel on detection, evaluation and treatment of high blood cholesterol in adults.** *Arch Intern Med* 1988, 148:36–69.
Recent pronouncement on the definition, detection and management of hypercholesterolaemia in the US population.

7. SNIDERMAN A, SHAPIRO S, MARPOLE D, SKINNER B, TENG B, KWITEROVICH PO: **Association of coronary atherosclerosis with hyperapobetalipoproteinemia [increased protein but normal cholesterol levels in human low density (β) lipoproteins].** *Proc Natl Acad Sci USA* 1980, 77:604–608.
The first description of the occurrence of hyperapoβlipoproteinaemia in patients with coronary disease, many of whom had LDL-apoB levels in the type II range despite being normocholesterolaemic.

8. UTERMANN G, HEES M, STEINMETZ A: **Polymorphism of apolipoprotein E and occurrence of dysbetalipoproteinaemia in man.** *Nature* 1977, 269:604–607.
The first description that type III hyperlipoproteinaemia was associated with an absence of the normal form of apoE, and that the latter is a polymorphic protein.

9. ZANNIS VI, BRESLOW JL: **Human very low density lipoprotein apolipoprotein E isoprotein polymorphism is explained by genetic variation and post-translational modification.** *Biochemistry* 1981, 20:1033–1041.
First demonstration that apoE is inherited at a single locus with three commonly occurring alleles and that type III hyperlipoproteinaemia is associated with homozygous inheritance of what the authors termed the ε4 allele, now termed ε2 (see [10]).

10. ZANNIS VI, BRESLOW JL, UTERMANN G, MAYLEY RW, WEISGRABER KH, HAVEL RJ, GOLDSTEIN JL, BROWN MS, SCHONFELD G, HAZZARD WR, BLUM C: **Proposed nomenclature of apoE isoproteins, apoE genotypes and phenotypes.** *J Lipid Res* 1982, 23:911–914.
Consensus report which reconciled the Utermann and Breslow systems of nomenclature.

11. HAVEL RJ: **Familial dysbetalipoproteinemia. New aspects of pathogenesis and diagnosis.** *Med Clin N Am* 1982, 66:441–454.
A useful review article which includes data on the frequency of apoE phenotypes and the biochemical changes responsible for the different phenotypes.

12. WARNICK GR, MAYFIELD C, ALBERS JJ, HAZZARD WR: **Gel isoelectric focusing method for specific diagnosis of familial hyperlipoproteinemia type 3.** *Clin Chem* 1979, 25:279–284.
A description of the standard method used to undertake apoE phenotyping.

4

13.   ORDOVAS JM, LITWACK-KLEIN L, WILSON PWF, SCHAEFER MM, SCHAEFER EJ: **Apolipoprotein E isoform phenotyping methodology and population frequency with identification of apoE1 and apoE5 isoforms.** *J Lipid Res* 1987, 28:371–380.
Description of a miniaturized method of determining apoE phenotypes with data on the frequency of both commonly occurring and rarer patterns in over 1000 subjects.

14.   HAVEKES LM, DE KNIJFF P, BEISIEGEL U, HAVINGA J, SMIT M, KLASEN E: **A rapid micromethod for apolipoprotein E phenotyping directly in serum.** *J Lipid Res* 1987, 28:455–463.
Description of a novel method of apoE phenotyping which avoids the need for ultracentrifugation by using immunoblotting to identify apoE isoforms after isoelectric focusing of serum.

15.   UTERMANN G: **Apolipoprotein E morphism in health and disease.** *Am Heart J* 1987, 113:433–440.
A review article which examines the varying expression of apoE polymorphism in different countries and proposes a mechanistic explanation for the associated variations in cholesterol levels, based on differential rates of clearance of remnant particles according to apoE phenotype.

16.   BRESLOW JL: **Human apolipoprotein molecular biology and genetic variation.** *Annu Rev Biochem* 1985, 54:699–727.
A detailed review of the molecular genetics of apolipoproteins.

17.   POAPST M, UFFELMAN K, STEINER G: **The chromogenicity and quantitation of apoB and apoB-48 of human plasma lipoproteins on analytical SDS gel electrophoresis.** *Atherosclerosis* 1987, 65:75–88.
Use of SDS-PAGE to separate $apoB_{48}$ and $apoB_{100}$ and examination of the problems involved in quantitating the two forms of apoB.

18.   UTERMANN G, MENZEL HJ, KRAFT HG, DUBA HC, KEMMLER HG, SEITZ C: **Lp(a) glycoprotein phenotypes.** *J Clin Invest* 1987, 80:458–465.
First description of apo(a) polymorphism.

4

5 LIPIDS AND RELATED VARIABLES AS RISK FACTORS

5

Epidemiology of lipids in relation to coronary heart disease

Introduction
'Risk factor' is an epidemiological term denoting a clinical or biochemical marker associated with a statistically increased likelihood of having or developing disease. Statistical association does not prove causality and the significance of risk factors in relation to the pathogenesis of CHD has to be evaluated in conjunction with clinical, genetic, experimental and pathological evidence. The evidence that hypercholesterolaemia due to an increase in LDL plays a causal role in atherogenesis is strong, whereas the precise mechanism involved in the inverse relationship between HDL cholesterol and CHD

remains to be determined. HDL could, for example, influence thrombogenesis rather than the atherosclerotic process *per se*. The three main lines of epidemiological evidence on which the lipid hypothesis is based are outlined below.

Geographic variation

The frequency of CHD varies widely between different populations, the age-standardized annual death rate from this cause in men in Scotland and Finland being around 435 per 100 000 compared with 64 per 100 000 in Japan (Table 5.1). The Seven Countries Study [1] showed close correlations between the incidence of CHD in men aged 40–59 and the proportion whose serum cholesterol exceeded 6.5 mmol/l, which ranged from 7% in Japan to 56% in Finland. Additional evidence suggested that these variations in serum cholesterol were largely attributable to differences in the ratio of saturated : unsaturated fats, including monounsaturates, in the national diet. The likelihood that contrasting dietary habits were responsible for the differences in both serum cholesterol and CHD is strengthened by the increase in both which occurred in Japanese who emigrated to the USA.

Table 5.1. Age-standardized death rates from ischaemic heart disease in males per 100 000 (World Health Organization Health Statistics Annual, 1984).

Scotland	436	Norway	306
Finland	434	West Germany	257
Ireland	387	Netherlands	253
New Zealand	378	Bulgaria	245
Sweden	377	Austria	245
Czechoslovakia	368	Belgium	196
England & Wales	360	Romania	191
Denmark	356	Italy	179
Australia	353	Greece	122
USA	348	Yugoslavia	118
Hungary	341	France	112
Canada	325	Japan	64

Case–control studies

These studies compare risk factors in individuals with clinical or angiographic evidence of past or present CHD and control subjects free from overt manifestations of this disorder. Such studies are inevitably open to bias in that there are several variables which could alter risk factors after CHD has become manifest, notably the changes in life-style which often occur after a myocardial infarct (MI) and also the effects of anti-anginal drugs. However, such studies have provided important information on the frequency of hyperlipidaemia both in patients with CHD and in their first-degree relatives. In Seattle over 30% of 500 MI survivors were hyperlipidaemic at 3 months and family studies showed that 20% of those below the age of 60 had a genetic basis for their hyperlipidaemia [2,3]. Several other case–control studies have also suggested that the younger the patient, the higher the frequency of hyperlipidaemia.

Prospective surveys

These provide important information about the relative strength and independence of risk factors as predictors of future disease in apparently healthy individuals. The most famous of all these surveys is the Framingham Study which started in 1949 and has been going ever since. Originally just over 5000 persons were examined and their subsequent incidence of CHD was determined [4]. By this means it was discovered that the likelihood of future CHD was markedly increased in those who initially had hypercholesterolaemia, hypertension or hyperglycaemia, or who smoked cigarettes, especially in those who had two or three of these risk factors. Subsequent analyses included an assessment of lipoproteins as well as lipids and their predictive power at different ages. The whole concept of preventive cardiology is largely predicated on the data which have emanated from Framingham and, despite its small sample size, it is still regarded as the benchmark against which all other prospective studies are measured.

5

Individual risk factors

Total cholesterol

Plasma or serum cholesterol concentration has been shown to correlate with CHD in both case–control and prospective studies. Initially it was thought that there was a threshold level below which the risk of CHD reached a plateau, but recent data from the Multiple Risk Factor Intervention Trial (MRFIT) study suggest that the risk is more or less continuous over the whole range of serum cholesterol. This survey involved more than 360 000 men aged 35–57 who were followed up for 6 years, during which more than 2400 died from CHD [5]. As shown in Fig. 5.1 the risk of CHD rises appreciably when the serum cholesterol exceeds 6.5 mmol/l and even more steeply when it rises above 7.8 mmol/l. Lowest rates of CHD occurred in men with serum cholesterol below 5.2 mmol/l. The correlation between total cholesterol and CHD in Framingham became much weaker in both sexes after the age of 55.

LDL cholesterol and apoB

The correlation between total cholesterol and CHD is almost entirely due to the correlation between the latter and the concentration of LDL in plasma, whether expressed as the mass of S_f 0–20 particles or the concentration of LDL cholesterol [6]. This correlation persists after middle-age and is present

5

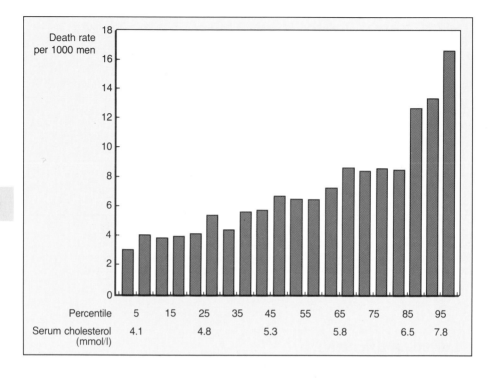

Fig. 5.1. Death rate from coronary heart disease in 360 000 men over 6 years according to percentile of serum cholesterol at time of screening. Adapted by permission [5].

in both men and women. Evidence for the causal nature of this association is reviewed in Chapter 6.

An alternative and relatively simple means of quantitating LDL is to measure LDL apoB. The advantage of this is that the mass of protein per LDL particle is constant whereas the amount of cholesterol carried by each particle can vary widely in both directions, high cholesterol : protein ratios being a feature of FH whereas low ratios are commonly seen in hypertriglyceridaemia. Thus measurement of apoB, which in most assays mainly reflects the apoB$_{100}$ in LDL, provides a better index of the number of LDL particles present in plasma than does measurement of LDL cholesterol. Comparison of these two variables as discriminants in a case–control study of subjects with and without angiographically proven coronary artery disease [7] shows less overlap between the two groups for apoB than for LDL cholesterol (Fig. 5.2). However, as yet there are no prospective data on whether apoB has more predictive power for CHD than does LDL cholesterol.

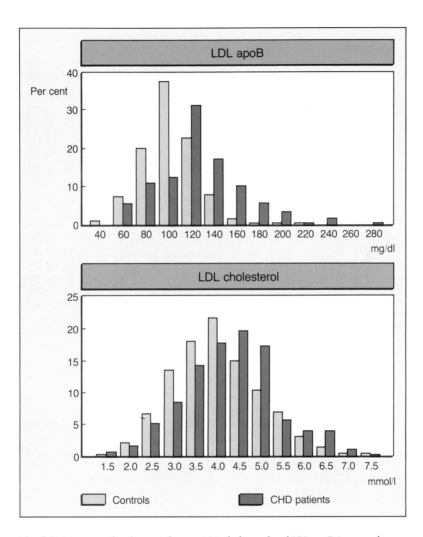

5

Fig. 5.2. Frequency distribution of serum LDL cholesterol and LDL apoB in control subjects and patients with coronary heart disease. Adapted by permission [7].

HDL cholesterol and apoA-I

The Framingham Study showed a strong, inverse correlation between HDL cholesterol and CHD in both sexes which was present on both univariate and multivariate analysis. The apparent protective effect of high concentrations of HDL cholesterol remained evident until the age of 80, whereas low values were associated with increased risk at all levels of total cholesterol, including those below 5.2 mmol/l [8]. Several other prospective studies have also shown an inverse relationship between HDL cholesterol and CHD. The opposing influences of total and HDL cholesterol have led to the use of various ratios as predictors of CHD risk, such as total : HDL cholesterol, LDL : HDL cholesterol and others, including the HDL ratio; this expresses the ratio of cholesterol in HDL to that in VLDL plus LDL as:

$$\frac{\text{HDL cholesterol}}{\text{Total} - \text{HDL cholesterol}}$$

The mechanism whereby HDL cholesterol influences CHD risk remains to be established but various hypotheses have been proposed, notably that HDL participates in the reverse transport of cholesterol from tissues and thereby reduces cholesterol accumulation in the arterial wall. An alternative possibility, particularly in view of its continuing influence on risk in later life, is that HDL or one of its components prevents the formation of thrombi on atheromatous plaques, for example by stabilization of prostacyclin in the vessel wall [9].

As with apoB and LDL there are also grounds for believing that quantitation of apoA-I gives a better index of HDL concentration than does measurement of HDL cholesterol. Serum apoA-I levels discriminate better than HDL cholesterol between individuals with and without coronary artery disease in case–control studies, as illustrated in Fig. 5.3, but prospective data are scanty.

Triglycerides and remnant particles

The role of fasting hypertriglyceridaemia as a risk factor is more controversial than the role of hypercholesterolaemia. Despite initial associations on univariate analysis, the correlation with CHD seldom remained significant on multivariate analysis when other confounding factors were taken into account, notably HDL cholesterol, with which triglycerides vary in a reciprocal manner. This has led to the suggestion that the association between raised triglycerides and CHD simply reflects the relationship between low HDL cholesterol and CHD [10].

Recently, however, there has been a trend towards accepting hypertriglyceridaemia as a risk factor in its own right. This has been due in part to the results of the Stockholm Prospective Study [11] and the Hammersmith Hospital Case–Control Study [7], in both of which triglyceride was an independent correlate of CHD on multivariate analysis. Also, reappraisal of data from the Framingham Study has shown that triglyceride was correlated with risk of CHD on multivariate analysis in women and also in men over 50 whose HDL cholesterol was below 1.03 mmol/l; this includes nine out of 10 hypertriglyceridaemic men in this age group [12].

There are several possible mechanisms whereby raised triglycerides could confer increased risk. It could be that they are simply a reflection of in-

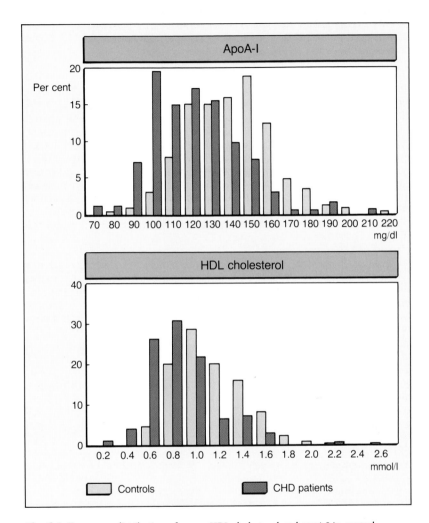

Fig. 5.3. Frequency distribution of serum HDL cholesterol and apoA-I in control subjects and patients with coronary heart disease. Adapted by permission [7].

creased numbers of remnant particles in plasma, which are thought to be atherogenic. This includes both increased concentrations of IDL in fasting plasma [13] and also of chylomicron remnants, determined by measuring the $apoB_{48} : apoB_{100}$ ratio in the d < 1.006 fraction of postprandial plasma [14]. Both types of abnormality have been described in patients with CHD.

Alternatively, hypertriglyceridaemia could simply be acting as a marker for the hypercoagulability that often accompanies it [15]. Smoking tends to aggravate both abnormalities, by impairing postprandial lipolysis and by raising fibrinogen levels in plasma.

Lp(a)

Lp(a) was discovered in 1963 by Berg as a genetic trait in human plasma. Subsequent workers described its physico-chemical properties and the association of high levels of Lp(a) with CHD. Angiographic studies suggest that the level of Lp(a) in plasma is a risk factor for disease of both native coronary vessels and bypass vein grafts, and is of the same order of magnitude as LDL cholesterol in this respect. The likelihood that Lp(a) and LDL are similarly atherogenic is suggested by their co-localization in atheromatous arteries and vein grafts. Although closely related to LDL structurally, the level of Lp(a) in plasma is thought to be regulated independently. However, it appears that the association between Lp(a) and CHD is dependent upon concomitant elevation of LDL cholesterol.

As mentioned previously, apo(a), a glycoprotein which exists in Lp(a) covalently linked to apoB$_{100}$, has considerable structural homology with plasminogen, both gene loci being closely linked on the long arm of chromosome 6. This has led to the suggestion that Lp(a) could have thrombogenic as well as atherogenic properties [16]. As discussed in the previous chapter, apo(a) is genetically polymorphic and Lp(a) levels in plasma are largely determined by which of several alleles at the apo(a) gene locus is inherited. This provides a genetic explanation for the observation that a raised level of Lp(a) could be substituted for a family history of premature CHD in discriminant function analysis of risk factors [17].

Age and sex

The absolute risk of CHD rises with age and is much greater at 65 than 35, as shown in Fig. 5.4. However, the relative risk increases with increasing serum cholesterol more steeply in 35-year-olds than in 65-year-olds. Thus the benefits of therapeutic intervention are likely to be greater if this is initiated sooner rather than later in life.

At any given level of serum cholesterol the risk of CHD in men is roughly three times that of women of comparable age (Fig. 5.5). For example, normotensive, non-smoking males aged 50 with a serum cholesterol of 4.8 mmol/l have roughly the same risk of developing CHD within 6 years as normotensive, non-smoking females of the same age with a serum cholesterol of 8.7 mmol/l. The relatively lower risk of CHD in women should be borne in mind when considering whether and how to intervene in the context of primary prevention. The precise mechanism for the greater protection enjoyed by females is uncertain but it probably reflects their having lower triglycerides

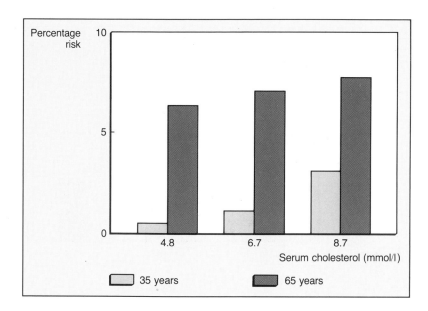

Fig. 5.4. Probability of developing coronary heart disease in 6 years in non-smoking, normotensive men aged 35 and 65 in the Framingham Study according to serum cholesterol at entry. Data from [18].

and higher HDL cholesterol levels than their male counterparts. This relative immunity tends to become less marked in females after the menopause.

Hypertension and smoking

The presence of hypertension more than doubles the risk of CHD at any given level of serum cholesterol and a similar but smaller increment is attributable to cigarette smoking. The co-existence of all three risk factors results in a multiplicative rather than an additive increase in risk, as illustrated in Fig. 5.6, such that the relative risk of CHD in hypercholesterolaemic, hypertensive smokers is nine times that of their normocholesterolaemic, normotensive, non-smoking contemporaries. Cessation of smoking eventually leads to a decrease in risk but hitherto treatment of hypertension has not resulted in any reduction in CHD, only a reduction in strokes. Conceivably this reflects the potentially adverse effects on serum lipids exerted by some of the commonly used antihypertensive drugs such as thiazide diuretics and beta blockers, which presumably offset the haemodynamic benefits of blood pressure reduction. However, certain other antihypertensives, such as angiotensin converting enzyme inhibitors and calcium antagonists, have a neutral effect on lipids. Cigarette smoking is associated with an increase in plasma fibrinogen

5

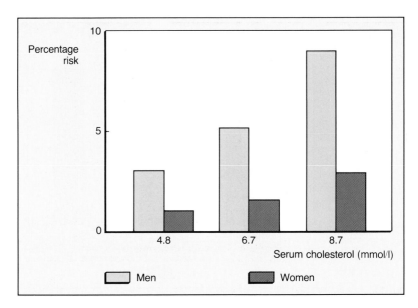

Fig. 5.5. Probability of developing coronary heart disease in 6 years in non-smoking, normotensive men and women age 50 in Framingham Study according to serum cholesterol at entry. Data from [18].

as well as with a reduction in HDL cholesterol, both changes being reversible within 1 year of cessation of the habit.

The relative risks of CHD in both sexes at various ages according to the presence or absence of hypertension and smoking, and also hyperglycaemia, based on the Framingham data, were published in tabulated form in 1973 [18]. Subsequent modification of these data to include HDL cholesterol led to the development of a multivariate risk equation [19]. However, even when all the conventional risk factors are taken into account this explains only 50% of the variability in risk of CHD. Predictability of CHD might be improved to some extent by inclusion of newer risk factors such as apoB, apoA-I, Lp(a) and fibrinogen. However, it is probable that other, hitherto unrecognized, risk factors exist which reflect the response of the arterial wall to atherogenic or thrombogenic influences, such as variations in endothelial permeability, macrophage function and fibrinolytic activity.

Corneal arcus and xanthelasma

The presence of a corneal arcus before the age of 60 is often a sign of hyper-cholesterolaemia. It also tends to occur more frequently in smokers than in

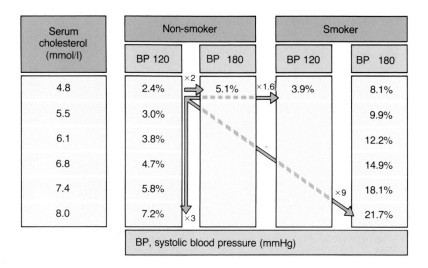

Fig. 5.6. Probability of developing coronary heart disease in 8 years in 45-year-old men with normal electrocardiogram in Framingham Study according to serum cholesterol, blood pressure and smoking habits. Adapted by permission from Thompson, in *Biochemical Aspects of Human Disease* edited by Elkeles and Tavill. Oxford: Blackwell, 1983, pp 85–123).

non-smokers. It reflects deposition of lipoprotein lipids within the cornea and is virtually irreversible. In one study involving over 3000 men the presence of an arcus was associated with a significantly increased risk of CHD even after adjusting for serum cholesterol and smoking [20].

Xanthelasma is a less specific sign of hyperlipidaemia than corneal arcus and is quite often seen in normolipidaemic subjects. However, even in this situation subtle abnormalities such as a raised VLDL cholesterol or decreased HDL:LDL cholesterol ratio seem relatively common and the frequency of CHD is reported to be increased [21].

Although the existence of corneal arcus and xanthelasma sometimes indicates the presence of an underlying increase in serum lipids, such as occurs in familial hypercholesterolaemia (see Chapter 8), the fact that these signs can occur in normolipidaemic individuals suggests that they may also reflect increases in tissue permeability. An accompanying increase in vascular endothelial permeability could be the reason why corneal arcus and xanthelasma appear to be risk factors in their own right rather than just markers of hyperlipidaemia.

Genetic variation in plasma lipids

Introduction

A family history of premature CHD is common in individuals with that disorder and occurred, for example, in 32–57% of patients in two recent studies in Britain [7,17]. Among the various possible explanations is the likelihood of familial similarities in risk factors, either inherited or resulting from shared environmental influences. Parent-sibling and twin studies show a high degree of heritability for total cholesterol, LDL cholesterol, HDL cholesterol and for apoB and apoA-I. In contrast plasma triglyceride and VLDL concentrations are related more to variations between family members in body weight and smoking habits.

5

Recent reviews suggest that 50–60% of the variability in serum cholesterol between individuals in Western industrialized populations is attributable to genetic variation, the precise nature of which is poorly defined but is presumed to be largely polygenic [22,23]. In contrast, it used to be considered that variations in serum lipids between populations were chiefly determined by environmental differences, especially diet. To a large extent this still holds true but there is increasing realization that genetic differences play a contributory role, exemplified by ethnic variations in the distribution of apoE phenotypes. The effects on serum lipids of apoE polymorphism are relatively easy to study because the gene products of the different alleles can be identified in plasma, as discussed in Chapter 4. This is not so with certain other forms of genetic polymorphism where it is necessary to search for alterations in the gene itself, using the technique known as restriction fragment length polymorphism (RFLP) analysis.

Because there are a large number of genes which could play a role in the genesis of hyperlipidaemia it makes sense to focus on those most likely to be involved, the so-called 'candidate genes' [22]. These include the gene for the LDL receptor, the apoA-I/C-III/A-IV gene cluster, the apoB gene, the apoE gene and the genes which encode the key enzymes and transfer proteins involved in lipoprotein metabolism. DNA probes for all eight of the major apolipoprotein genes are now available and polymorphisms have been detected in all of them [24]. However, reported associations between specific polymorphisms and variations in plasma lipids and apoproteins have sometimes been inconsistent, with different groups of workers obtaining contradictory results. Also, association between certain polymorphisms and CHD has been reported, but often without any change in the plasma level of the risk factor encoded by the gene under study. Thus, analysis of RFLPs is still at the research stage and its clinical usefulness remains to be established.

A comprehensive and up-to-date description of RFLP analysis in relation to atherosclerosis can be obtained from the reviews already cited [22,24]. Here we will confine ourselves to a brief discussion of the relative contributions made by polymorphism of apoE and apoB to variations in serum cholesterol both within and between populations.

ApoE polymorphism

As discussed previously, there are three common alleles, $\varepsilon 2$, $\varepsilon 3$ and $\varepsilon 4$, which are inherited in a co-dominant manner. The relative frequency of these alleles varies between populations, the frequency of the commonest allele, $\varepsilon 3$, ranging from 0.88 in Singaporian Indians [25] to 0.77 in Caucasians [23]. The relative frequency of the $\varepsilon 2$ allele is lowest in Japan (0.02) and highest in France (0.13). The $\varepsilon 4$ allele is least common among the Chinese (0.06) but has a relative frequency of almost 0.23 in Finns. Measurement of serum cholesterol shows that in comparison with those carrying the 'normal' $\varepsilon 3$ allele, those with the $\varepsilon 2$ allele have a lower mean serum cholesterol whereas the opposite occurs in those with the $\varepsilon 4$ allele. Differences in the frequency of the $\varepsilon 2$ and $\varepsilon 4$ alleles contribute to differences in cholesterol levels between countries, although for each phenotype levels are higher among the Finns than among the Japanese, reflecting the overriding influence of diet.

5

It has been calculated that on average approximately 7% of the phenotypic variance of serum cholesterol between individuals is attributable to apoE polymorphism, largely due to differences in LDL cholesterol. The mechanism involved reflects the role of apoE as a ligand for the LDL receptor, and possibly the chylomicron remnant receptor, and its involvement in the conversion of IDL to LDL. Remnant particles containing $apoE_2$ are cleared abnormally slowly, because of defective binding of $apoE_2$ to the relevant receptors, and IDL conversion to LDL is also impaired. Consequently less cholesterol is taken up by the liver and LDL receptors are up-regulated, leading to a decreased concentration of LDL in plasma. In contrast $apoE_4$-bearing particles appeared to be cleared faster than normal, which leads to down-regulation of LDL receptors and a consequent increase in plasma LDL cholesterol. As reviewed elsewhere [23], there is evidence that persons with the $\varepsilon 4$ allele have an increased risk of CHD compared with those homozygous for $\varepsilon 3$, whereas those with the $\varepsilon 2$ allele are protected, unless they develop type III hyperlipoproteinaemia. The latter disorder together with the biochemical differences between the various isoforms of apoE are discussed in Chapter 9.

ApoB gene polymorphism

The large size and insolubility of apoB makes detection of polymorphism of the protein itself extremely difficult. However, now that the gene has been cloned it has become possible to subject it to RFLP analysis. At least eight different polymorphisms have been described so far [22]. One of these, the XbaI RFLP, has been reported to be associated with variations in LDL cholesterol and apoB in some studies [24] due, it is claimed, to altered catabolism of LDL. However, the mechanism involved is unclear since this particular RFLP does not change the amino acid sequence of apoB. Another group failed to find any association between XbaI RFLP and variations in serum cholesterol but did find such a relationship with the MspI and EcoRI RFLPs, both of which are associated with amino acid changes in the receptor-binding domain of apoB [26]. These authors suggested that approximately 3.5% of the variance in serum cholesterol might be explicable by these polymorphisms.

Genetic versus environmental variation

It has been estimated that 63% of the phenotypic variation in serum cholesterol is genetically determined, including the contributions made by apoB and apoE polymorphisms, whereas the remaining 37% is due to environmental influences such as diet [23]. By far the largest segment of the genetic component is attributed to residual polygenes, the nature of which remains largely speculative at present. However, it seems likely that included in that category are as yet undiscovered gene polymorphisms which influence LDL receptor activity and apoB synthesis. Monogenic disorders such as FH have a major effect on serum cholesterol in affected individuals but, because of their infrequency, exert relatively little influence on the overall variation within populations. The main determinant of the latter must surely be interaction between residual polygenes and non-genetic factors such as diet and physical activity. At present our ability to determine the respective contributions made by genetic and non-genetic factors to commonly recurring, non-monogenic forms of hyperlipidaemia is largely confined to the therapeutic trial of a lipid-lowering diet. Hopefully, more precise indices of the genetic component will eventually become available.

Annotated references

1.   KEYS A: Coronary heart disease in seven countries. *Circulation* 1970, 41 (suppl 1):I1–I21.
The Seven Countries Study of Ancel Keys and colleagues made a major contribution to establishing the link between diet, hypercholesterolaemia and CHD.

2.   GOLDSTEIN JL, HAZZARD WR, SCHROTT HG, BIERMAN EL, MOTULSKY AG: **Hyperlipidemia in coronary heart disease. I. Lipid levels in 500 survivors of myocardial infarction.** *J Clin Invest* 1973, 52:1533–1543.
This large study by Goldstein and colleagues helped establish the frequency of genetically determined forms of hyperlipidaemia in relation to CHD.

3.   GOLDSTEIN JL, SCHROTT HG, HAZZARD WR, BIERMAN EL, MOTULSKY AG: **Hyperlipidemia in coronary heart disease. II. Genetic analysis of lipid levels in 176 families and delineation of a new inherited disorder, combined hyperlipidemia.** *J Clin Invest* 1973, 52:1544–1568.
See [2].

4.   KANNEL WB, DAWBER TR, KAGAN A, REVOTSKIE N, STOKES J: **Factors of risk in the development of coronary heart disease — six year follow-up experience: the Framingham Study.** *Ann Intern Med* 1961, 55:33–50.
A description of some of the earlier data from Framingham.

5.   MARTIN MJ, HULLEY SB, BROWNER WS, KULLER LH, WENTWORTH D: **Serum cholesterol, blood pressure and mortality: implications from a cohort of 361 662 men.** *Lancet* 1986, ii:933–936.
This paper describes the largest sample of men ever followed prospectively to determine the incidence of CHD in relation to risk factors.

6.   KANNEL WB, GORDON T, CASTELLI WP: **Role of lipids and lipoprotein fractions in assessing atherogenesis. The Framingham Study.** *Prog Lipid Res* 1981, 20:339–348.
Another appraisal from Framingham, in this instance of the relationship between CHD risk and lipoproteins at different ages.

7.   BARBIR M, WILE D, TRAYNER I, ABER VR, THOMPSON GR: **High prevalence of hyper-triglyceridaemia and apolipoprotein abnormalities in coronary artery disease.** *Br Heart J* 1988, 60:397–403.
Case–control study of risk factors in almost 200 patients with CHD at the Hammersmith Hospital and over 500 controls at the British United Provident Association Medical Centre in London.

8.   CASTELLI WP, GARRISON RJ, WILSON PWF, ABBOTT RD, KALOUSDIAN S, KANNEL WB: **Incidence of coronary heart disease and lipoprotein cholesterol levels.** *JAMA* 1986, 256:2835–2838.
Twelve years' follow-up data from Framingham confirming the inverse correlation between HDL cholesterol and CHD.

9.   YUI Y, AOYAMA T, MORISHITA H, TAKAHASHI M, TAKATSU Y, KAWAI C: **Serum prostacyclin stabilizing factor is identical to apolipoprotein A-I (apoA-I).** *J Clin Invest* 1988, 82:803–807.
Demonstration that HDL binds prostacyclin and thereby prolongs its half-life, this action being mediated by apoA-I.

10.   HULLEY SB, ROSENMAN RH, BAWOL RD, BRAND RJ: **Epidemiology as a guide to clinical decisions. The association between triglyceride and coronary heart disease.** *N Engl J Med* 1980, 302:1383–1389.
Data from the Western Collaborative prospective study which questions the independence of the epidemiological association between triglycerides and CHD.

11.   CARLSON LA, BÖTTIGER LE: **Risk factors for ischaemic heart disease in men and women. Results of the 19-year follow-up of the Stockholm Prospective Study.** *Acta Med Scand* 1985, 218:207–211.
A prospective study of 3000 men and 3000 women shows that triglycerides are an independent risk factor for death from myocardial infarction.

12.   CASTELLI WP: **The triglyceride issue: a view from Framingham.** *Am Heart J* 1986, 112:432–437.

5

Re-appraisal by Castelli of relationship between triglycerides and CHD in Framingham. He concludes that it is an independent risk factor after all, except in men with a normal HDL cholesterol.

13.   STEINER G, SCHWARTZ L, SHUMAK S, POAPST M: **The association of increased levels of intermediate density lipoproteins with smoking and with coronary artery disease.** *Circulation* 1987, **75**:124–130.
Angiographic study showing independent correlation between IDL and coronary atherosclerosis.

14.   SIMONS LA, DWYER T, SIMONS J, BERNSTEIN L, MOCK P, POONIA NS, BALASUBRAMANIAM S, BARON D, BRANSON J, MORGAN J, ROY P: **Chylomicrons and chylomicron remnants in coronary artery disease: a case-control study.** *Atherosclerosis* 1987, **65**:181–189.
Case–control study showing increased postprandial ratio of $apoB_{48}:apoB_{100}$, an index of chylomicrons and remnants, in patients with angiographically proven coronary disease.

15.   SIMPSON HCR, MANN JI, MEADE TW, CHAKRABARTI R, STIRLING Y, WOOLF L: **Hypertriglyceridaemia and hypercoagulability.** *Lancet* 1983, i:786–790.
Study showing that patients with type IV hyperlipoproteinaemia had higher levels of factor X and fibrinogen and lower fibrinolytic activity than controls.

16.   BROWN MS, GOLDSTEIN JL: **Teaching old dogmas new tricks.** *Nature* 1987, **330**:113–114.
Leading article which suggests that the close homology between Lp(a) and plasminogen discovered by McLean *et al.* may provide a link between the lipid insudative and thrombogenic theories of atherogenesis.

17.   DURRINGTON PN, ISHOLA M, HUNT L, ARROL S: **Apolipoproteins(a), AI and B and parental history in men with early onset ischaemic heart disease.** *Lancet* 1988, i:1070–1073.
Case–control study showing that much of the familial predisposition to CHD appears to be due to increased levels of Lp(a) in plasma.

18.   AMERICAN HEART ASSOCIATION: *Coronary Risk Handbook. Estimating Risk of Coronary Heart Disease in Daily Practice.* American Heart Association, 1973, pp 1–50.
Tables showing relation between serum cholesterol, blood pressure, smoking, glucose intolerance and ECG abnormalities and risk of future CHD, based on Framingham data.

19.   WILSON PWF, CASTELLI WP, KANNEL WB: **Coronary risk prediction in adults (the Framingham Heart Study).** *Am J Cardiol* 1987, **59**:91G–94G.
Updated method of calculating risk of CHD in the form of a multivariate logistic function which includes HDL cholesterol and is suitable for use in programmable calculators and computers.

20.   ROSENMAN RH, BRAND RJ, SHOLTZ RI, JENKINS CD: **Relation of corneal arcus to cardiovascular risk factors and the incidence of coronary disease.** *N Engl J Med* 1974, **291**:1322–1324.
Frequency of corneal arcus studied in relation to age, serum cholesterol, cigarette smoking and CHD over an $8\frac{1}{2}$-year period of follow-up.

5

21.   WATANABE A, YOSHIMURA A, WAKASUGI T, TATAMI R, UEDA K, UEDA R, HABA T, KAMETANI T, KOIZUMI J, ITO S, OHTA M, MIYAMOTO S, MABUCHI H, TAKEDA R: **Serum lipids, lipoprotein lipids and coronary heart disease in patients with xanthelasma palpebrarum.** *Atherosclerosis* 1981, **38**:283–290.
Analysis of VLDL, LDL and HDL cholesterol concentrations in a small number of patients with xanthelasma, some of whom had normal total cholesterol and triglyceride, including several with CHD.

22.   LUSIS AJ: **Genetic factors affecting blood lipoproteins: the candidate gene approach.** *J Lipid Res* 1988, **29**:397–429.
Comprehensive and recent review of the molecular biological approach to the genetic basis of atherosclerosis, with over 300 references.

23.   DAVIGNON J, GREGG RE, SING CF: **Apolipoprotein E polymorphism and atherosclerosis.** *Arteriosclerosis* 1988, **8**:1–21.
Detailed analysis of the data of Utermann and others of the relationship between apoE polymorphism, blood lipids and predisposition to CHD.

24.   HUMPHRIES SE: **DNA polymorphisms of the apolipoprotein genes — their use in the investigation of the genetic component of hyperlipidaemia and atherosclerosis.** *Atherosclerosis* 1988, **72**:89–108.
Detailed review of the role of RFLP analysis in relation to genetically determined hyperlipidaemia.

25.   UTERMANN G: **Apolipoprotein polymorphism and multifactorial hyperlipidaemia.** *J Inher Metab Dis* 1988, (suppl 1):74–86.
Useful review of genetic polymorphism of apoE and Lp(a).

26.   RAJPUT-WILLIAMS J, KNOTT TJ, WALLIS SC, SWEETNAM P, YARNELL J, COX N, BELL GI, MILLER NE, SCOTT J: **Variation of apolipoprotein-B gene is associated with obesity, high blood cholesterol levels, and increased risk of coronary heart disease.** *Lancet* 1988, **ii**:1442–1446.
Assessment of contribution of three apoB gene polymorphisms to variations in serum cholesterol in the Caerphilly Study.

5

6 PATHOGENESIS OF ATHEROSCLEROSIS

6

Introduction

The terms atheroma and atherosclerosis are derived from the Greek words, *athere* meaning gruel, *oma* meaning a mass, and *skleros* meaning hard. They aptly describe the nature of the lesions which characterize this degenerative disease of blood vessels, currently the commonest cause of death and disability in most Westernized countries.

Causal role of risk factors

Atherosclerosis is defined as a variable combination of changes in the intima (inner lining) of arteries consisting of the focal accumulation of lipids, other blood constituents and fibrous tissue, accompanied by changes in the media (middle layer) of the vessel wall. These features are the result of interaction between the structural and metabolic properties of the arterial wall, components of the blood and haemodynamic forces [1].

Two factors which have a major bearing on the occurrence of atherosclerosis are its correlation with raised plasma lipids and the influence of blood pressure. Thus the condition seldom affects individuals whose serum cholesterol is less than 4 mmol/l, as is common among the Japanese, nor does it affect veins unless these are exposed to arterial levels of blood pressure, as happens when saphenous veins are used to bypass diseased coronary arteries. Other determinants of atherosclerosis are age and sex, as illustrated in Fig. 6.1, which also influence, respectively, the concentration of cholesterol in plasma and its distribution between LDL and HDL.

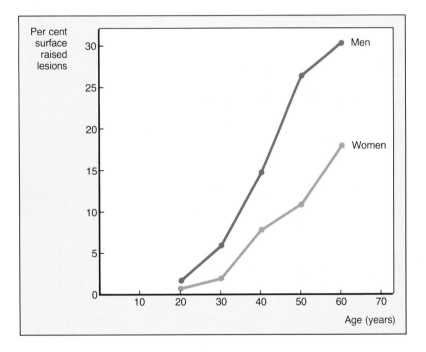

Fig. 6.1. Mean extent of intimal surface involved by raised lesions in the coronary arteries in relation to age and sex. Adapted by permission of the American Heart Association, Inc., from McGill, *Arteriosclerosis* 1984, 4:443–451.

The correlation between raised LDL levels and atherosclerosis not only holds true for cholesterol but also applies to apoB. An increased prevalence of atherosclerotic disorders has been reported in individuals with increased levels of LDL apoB, despite relatively normal levels of LDL cholesterol. This apparent paradox reflects overproduction of LDL particles which are smaller and denser than normal and depleted in cholesterol ester. Such particles penetrate the arterial wall more easily than larger LDL particles, such as occur in FH. Retention of LDL occurs as a result of electrostatic interaction between apoB and glycosaminoglycans, or its hydrophobic interaction with elastin, both being connective tissue constituents of the vessel wall. Recent studies suggest that Lp(a) has even greater affinity than LDL for glycosaminoglycans [2].

HDL particles do not undergo these interactions but instead have the ability to take up free cholesterol from other lipoproteins and various tissues including, it is assumed, the arterial wall. This cholesterol subsequently undergoes esterification by LCAT and is then conveyed back into the bloodstream via the lymphatics. Thus the net flux of cholesterol into and out of the arterial wall is influenced by the ratio of LDL and HDL particles in the interstitial fluid. Haemodynamic factors help determine the localization of atherosclerosis to particular sites by differentially influencing the influx and efflux of these lipoprotein particles.

The epidemiological delineation of risk factors has not only provided a valuable means of identifying those at increased risk of developing CHD, but has also contributed to an understanding of the pathogenesis of atherosclerosis. Coronary atherosclerosis is the most serious form of the disease and contributes vastly to premature death and disability in Britain where death rates from CHD are currently among the highest in the world. However, it is important to distinguish between CHD and coronary atherosclerosis, in that the former reflects the combined consequences of the latter and secondary thrombotic changes. Thus if a silent lesion in a major branch of a coronary artery develops a small fissure, it may then become acutely occluded by a superimposed thrombus, which can result in the sudden death of a previously asymptomatic individual [3]. The third of the major risk factors, smoking, probably exerts its main effects on the thrombogenic component of CHD, by increasing fibrinogen levels. The remainder of this chapter will focus on the pathogenesis of atherosclerosis rather than on the thrombotic aspects of CHD.

6

Pathology

Introduction
The characteristic lesion of atherosclerosis is the fibrous plaque, which consists of a cap of smooth muscle cells and fibrous tissue covered by a layer of endothelium, and a core containing yellowish lipid [4]. These features are illustrated diagrammatically in Fig. 6.2. In fatal cases, the lumen of at least one major branch of a coronary artery, more usually two or three, is narrowed to less than 25% of its original diameter by such plaques [5]. Fibrous tissue is the main constituent but up to 45% of the lesion consists of lipid, mainly cholesterol. This cholesterol is derived almost entirely from the blood and not from local synthesis.

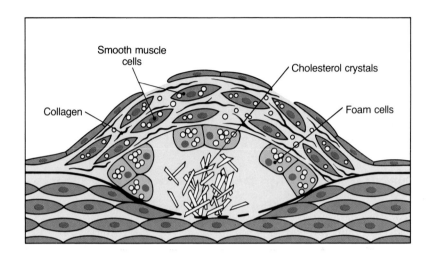

Fig. 6.2. Diagrammatic representation of an atheromatous plaque showing outer cap containing collagen and smooth muscle cells, and inner core containing foam cells and extracellular cholesterol crystals. Adapted by permission from *Heart Disease: A Textbook of Cardiovascular Medicine* edited by Braunwald. Saunders, 1980.

Smith and Slater [6] showed a close correlation between the concentration of LDL cholesterol in aortic intima *post mortem* and the serum cholesterol level in blood taken during the week before death. Other studies have shown correlations between the extent and severity of coronary atherosclerosis and serum cholesterol concentrations measured up to 9 years prior to death [7]. The importance of hypercholesterolaemia, especially when due to an increase in LDL, as a causal factor in atherosclerosis is underlined by the latter's severity in individuals with FH, in whom LDL levels are two to four times higher than normal throughout life. In contrast, individuals with hyperαlipoproteinaemia, who have an increase in HDL cholesterol, are not at increased risk of CHD. On the contrary, they appear to enjoy some degree of protection against that disorder.

Response to injury hypothesis
In 1976 Ross and Harker [8] proposed a modification of Virchow's original 'response to injury' hypothesis in which they stressed the importance of endothelial damage as the initiating event in atherogenesis. Injury, they suggested, could stem from various causes, including hypercholesterolaemia, and led to entry of platelets into the arterial wall. This event was followed by proliferation of medial smooth muscle cells and their migration into the intima.

Subsequent studies showed this to be due to the effects of a platelet-derived growth factor (PDGF) on smooth muscle cells.

Recently Ross has put forward a revised version of this hypothesis, based upon evidence from electron micrographic studies in monkeys with diet-induced hypercholesterolaemia [9]. Such studies show that within 2 weeks of starting the diet, clusters of monocytes become attached to the endothelial surface of arteries. These monocytes subsequently penetrate beneath the endothelium, accumulate lipid and turn into foam cells, that is to say macrophages containing large amounts of esterified cholesterol. For many years these foam cells were thought to be derived from smooth muscle cells but recent evidence supports their monocytic origin [10].

After several months of hypercholesterolaemia, the endothelium over collections of foam cells, visible to the naked eye as fatty streaks, starts to retract and in some instances exposes the underlying macrophages to the circulation. This results in adherence of platelets, with mural thrombus formation, and leads to hyperplasia of smooth muscle cells and the eventual conversion of a fatty streak into a proliferative lesion. A similar sequence of events is observed in Watanabe heritable hyperlipidaemic (WHHL) rabbits, which have a genetically determined form of hypercholesterolaemia due to a deficiency of LDL receptors, analogous to FH in humans.

6

It has been shown that endothelial cells in culture release several growth factors, including one resembling PDGF, which exert a chemotactic effect on monocytes and a stimulatory effect on the growth of smooth muscle cells. Attachment of monocytes to the endothelium is mediated by the influence of hypercholesterolaemia on the monocytes themselves as well as on endothelial cells. Smooth muscle cells possess receptors for PDGF and respond to stimulation by multiplying and producing connective tissue.

PDGF has been partly purified and has a molecular weight of roughly 30 000 [11]. It, or similar growth factors, can be secreted not only by platelets but also by endothelial cells and macrophages. Endothelial injury plays a key role by initiating a series of events which result in humoral promotion of the growth of smooth muscle cells and fibroblasts. The initial injury can occur in several ways, including haemodynamic sheer stresses ('wear and tear'), toxic damage mediated by cigarette smoking (carbon monoxide), immune complexes, viruses or homocysteine, and increased levels of LDL *per se*. The subsequent series of events which eventually results in a proliferative lesion is illustrated in Fig. 6.3.

Role of macrophages
Throughout this chapter stress has been laid on the causal role of hypercholesterolaemia due to an increase in LDL in the aetiology of atherosclerosis. Furthermore, it should also be evident that the cholesterol ester loaded macrophage, or foam cell, is the most distinctive histological feature of an

6

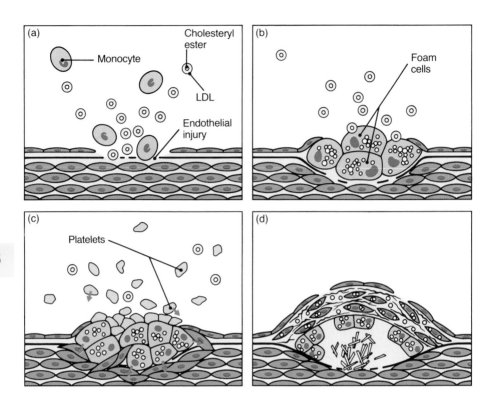

Fig. 6.3. Response to injury hypothesis of atherogenesis. Arrows indicate growth factors.

atheromatous plaque. The inference is that monocyte-derived macrophages become foam cells by ingesting, hydrolysing and re-esterifying the cholesterol ester present in LDL. Paradoxically, however, although monocytes possess LDL receptors, these become down-regulated as soon as the cholesterol content of the cell increases and it has so far proved impossible to transform monocytes into foam cells simply by exposing them to native LDL *in vitro*.

Monocytes possess not only LDL receptors but also receptors for various forms of modified LDL, including acetyl LDL. Unlike LDL receptors, acetyl LDL receptors are not down-regulated by accumulation of cholesterol within macrophages. It is most unlikely that LDL is ever acetylated *in vivo* but a chemical reaction which might well occur is oxidative modification.

It is known that *in vitro* incubation of LDL with cultured endothelial cells, smooth muscle cells or macrophages leads to peroxidation of LDL phospholipids, resulting in conversion of lecithin to lysolecithin and partial degradation of apoB [12]. The oxidatively modified LDL is taken up avidly by macrophages via their acetyl LDL receptors but it remains to be shown whether this process occurs *in vivo*. Circumstantial evidence that it does is based on the beneficial effect of anti-oxidants in preventing foam cell formation *in vitro* and preventing progression of experimentally induced atheroma. Additional evidence comes from the presence in atheromatous lesions of ceroid, the alcohol-insoluble remnant of oxidized LDL which is resistant to lysosomal digestion by macrophages [13]. This poses the intriguing question whether macrophages perform a vital scavenger function at sites of endothelial damage in the arterial wall by taking up and digesting LDL or whether their presence there leads to the accumulation of lipid-laden foam cells which release growth factors and thus promote migration of smooth muscle cells from the media, with a consequent increase in collagen formation. The answer presumably depends upon how much LDL accumulates at the site of intimal damage. Whether or not this is manageable will in turn depend upon plasma LDL levels and the functional efficiency of the reverse cholesterol transport pathway.

6

Factors influencing progression and regression

Introduction
Hitherto, most attempts to induce regression of atheroma have been based on the premise that reduction of hypercholesterolaemia should eventually lead to depletion of the cholesterol content of plaques. This is a slow process, especially when much of the cholesterol is crystalline and extracellular rather than esterified and within foam cells, the latter form being more amenable to mobilization. Determining the precise role of HDL in this process is hampered by lack of a suitable animal model.

Experimental evidence
Atheroma can be produced experimentally in a number of animal species by diet-induced hypercholesterolaemia. Withdrawal of the dietary stimulus and return of the plasma cholesterol to basal levels results in the gradual regression of the atheromatous lesions that developed during the period of hypercholesterolaemia. Some of the most convincing data have come from studies undertaken in primates, as reviewed by Wissler [14]. As a rule, plasma cholesterol levels in non-human primates must be reduced to 4 mmol/l or less for 12–18 months to achieve regression of lesions induced by 18 months of hypercholesterolaemia. The pathological changes that occur during regression include a decrease in the size and lipid content of the atheromatous plaque, fewer foam cells and a smaller necrotic area in the core of the lesion, and an increase in the cell density and collagen content of the fibrous cap (Fig. 6.4). The increase in collagen is slow to diminish and never returns

completely to basal levels. Thus, although regression results in a widening of the arterial lumen, the vessel wall becomes fibrosed and may fail to dilate normally in response to physiological stimuli [15].

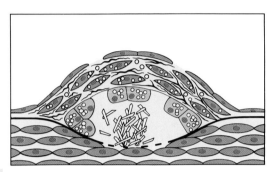 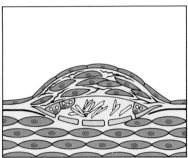

6

Fig. 6.4. Histological changes in experimentally induced atherosclerotic plaque before (left) and after (right) 18 months of cholesterol-lowering therapy. Adapted by permission [14].

Kinetic considerations

All regression regimens are based on the premise that mobilization of the cholesterol component of atheromatous plaques requires the creation of a reverse concentration gradient between the arterial wall and plasma. Assuming that at least 25% of an atheromatous plaque is cholesterol, a significant reduction in the cholesterol content of the plaque could result in a functionally significant improvement in blood flow in a critically stenosed (> 75%) coronary artery, as illustrated in Fig. 6.5. Thus, it is important to consider the physico-chemical state of cholesterol within atheromatous plaques and the speed with which this turns over.

The turnover time of cholesterol in human atheromatous plaques is approximately 1½–3 years, far slower than its rate of turnover in most other tissues, including the cutaneous or tendon xanthomata of hypercholesterolaemic patients [16]. In advanced plaques, the proportion of unesterified cholesterol is twice that found in xanthomata, in which most of the cholesterol is esterified. High concentrations of unesterified cholesterol tend to crystallize and the turnover rate of cholesterol crystals deep in the plaque is much slower than that of esterified cholesterol in the more superficial layers [17]. Most of the cholesterol ester is within macrophages, or foam cells, and a reduction in the number of these cells during the early stages of regression is accompanied by a paradoxical increase in cholesterol crystals. Because of this and the accompanying increase in collagen content, regression of advanced lesions is likely to be both slow and incomplete.

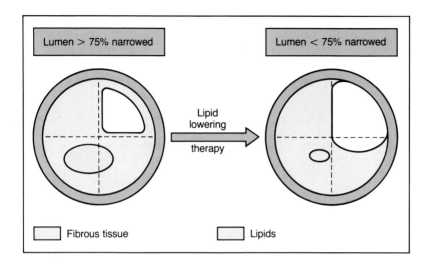

Fig. 6.5. Diagrammatic representation of effects of lipid-lowering therapy on lipid content and degree of stenosis of atherosclerotic artery. Adapted by permission [5].

Angiographic data

Numerous studies have shown a relation between the severity of angiographically assessed coronary artery disease and hyperlipidaemia, as judged by the earliness of age of onset of symptoms, the multiplicity of vessels involved, and the tendency for lesions to progress. Angiographic abnormalities are associated more closely with hypercholesterolaemia than with hypertriglyceridaemia and correlate inversely with the ratio between HDL cholesterol, especially its HDL_2 subfraction, and LDL cholesterol. Increases in LDL cholesterol and decreases in HDL cholesterol are each independently associated with the severity of disease and the tendency for lesions to progress is inversely correlated with the HDL:LDL cholesterol ratio. Histological and angiographic studies in patients who have undergone coronary artery bypass grafting (CABG) show evidence of atheromatous involvement in the majority of saphenous vein grafts within 10 years, these changes too being correlated with increased levels of LDL and decreased levels of HDL.

Angiographic evidence of regression of human atherosclerosis is limited. A review of this topic cited 32 instances out of a total of 143 patients but these were all drawn from anecdotal reports or uncontrolled studies [18]. Computer-assisted analysis of coronary angiograms shows that untreated lesions are three times more likely to progress than regress over a period of 18 months, the propensity to progression being even greater in hyperlipidaemic individuals [19].

Recently, however, it has become apparent that effective lipid-lowering therapy can slow the rate of progression or even induce regression of atheromatous lesions. As shown in Fig. 6.6, moderate reduction of LDL cholesterol (from 5.7 to 4.6 mmol/l) and a modest increase in the HDL:LDL ratio (from 0.20 to 0.26) by treatment with cholestyramine in patients with type II hyperlipoproteinaemia were associated with a significant reduction in the percentage of coronary lesions which progressed [20] whereas the more marked reductions in LDL cholesterol (from 4.1 to 2.5 mmol/l) and increases in the HDL:LDL ratio (from 0.27 to 0.59) achieved in the Cholesterol Lowering Atherosclerosis Study (CLAS) trial by a combination of colestipol and nicotinic acid resulted in a significant increase in lesions which regressed [21]. Both were double-blind trials but they differed in the greater severity of hypercholesterolaemia in the type II trial and the lumping together of lesions of native vessels and bypass grafts in the CLAS trial, which investigated only patients who had previously undergone CABG. Nevertheless these findings, when taken together with those of earlier uncontrolled trials of diet or diet and drugs, do suggest that, as in non-human primates, so also in man the anatomical lesions of atherosclerosis can be favourably influenced by lipid-lowering therapy. This being so, it remains to be shown whether it is more cost-effective to attempt to reverse established disease or to try to pre-empt its development in those at risk. The results of several primary and secondary prevention trials suggest that both approaches reduce morbidity and mortality from CHD, as reviewed in chapter 14.

6

Annotated references

1.   GETZ GS, VESSELINOVITCH D, WISSLER RW: **A dynamic pathology of atherosclerosis.** *Am J Med* 1969, 46:657–673.
Slightly dated but useful review of the principles involved in understanding the causation of atherosclerosis.

2.   BIHARI-VARGA M, GRUBER E, ROTHENEDER M, ZECHNER R, KOSTNER GM: **Interaction of lipoprotein (a) and low density lipoprotein with glycosoaminoglycans from human aorta.** *Arteriosclerosis* 1988, 8:851–857.
Comparison of binding to aortic glycosaminoglycans of LDL and Lp(a).

3.   DAVIES MJ, THOMAS A: **Thrombosis and acute coronary artery lesions in sudden cardiac ischaemic death.** *N Engl J Med* 1984, 310:1137–1140.
Major study involving post-mortem injection of coronary arteries which demonstrates the importance of plaque fissuring as a cause of fatal coronary thrombosis.

4.   PEARSON TA, KRAMER EC, SOLEZ K, HEPTINSTALL RH: **The human atherosclerotic plaque.** *Am J Pathol* 1977, 86:657–664.
Review of the main theories of the pathogenesis of atherosclerosis, including Benditt's monoclonal hypothesis.

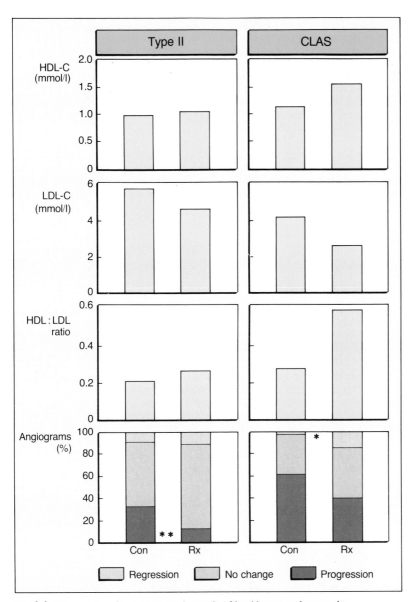

6

Fig. 6.6. Comparison of two angiographic trials of lipid-lowering therapy, the National Heart Lung and Blood Institute type II coronary intervention study and the Cholesterol-Lowering Atherosclerosis Study (CLAS), showing the effects of diet plus placebo (Con) versus diet plus drugs (Rx) on HDL cholesterol, LDL cholesterol, HDL:LDL ratio and angiographic change. *$P = 0.002$; **$P = 0.02$.

5.   ROBERTS WC: **The status of the coronary arteries in fatal ischemic heart disease.** *Cardiovasc Clin* 1975, 7:1–24.
Detailed description of post-mortem findings in fatal CHD, including the frequent occurrence of fibrous plaques causing >75% stenosis of one or more major vessels.

6.   SMITH E, SLATER RS: **Relationship between low density lipoprotein in aortic intima and serum lipid levels.** *Lancet* 1972, i:463.
Classic study involving the immunological measurement of LDL in the aortic wall at postmortem examination and its correlation with the ante-mortem concentration of serum cholesterol in 21 individuals.

7.   FEINLEIB M, KANNEL WB, TEDESCHI CG, LANDAU TK, GARRISON RJ: **The relation of antemortem characteristics to cardiovascular findings at necropsy.** *Atherosclerosis* 1979, 34:145–157.
Careful analysis of the extent and degree of coronary atherosclerosis in 127 fatalities from the Framingham Study in relation to serum cholesterol values measured up to 9 years previously.

8.   ROSS R, HARKER L: **Hyperlipidemia and atherosclerosis.** *Science* 1976, 193:1094–1100.
Important article which proposed that endothelial damage is the crucial initiating event in atherogenesis and that subsequent changes are a response to such injury.

9.   ROSS R: **The pathogenesis of atherosclerosis — an update.** *N Engl J Med* 1986, 314:488–500.
Revision of the original 'response to injury' concept which takes account of new knowledge of the role of PDGF and other growth factors.

10.   AQEL NM, BALL RY, WALDMANN H, MITCHINSON MJ: **Monocytic origin of foam cells in human atherosclerotic plaques.** *Atherosclerosis* 1984, 53:265–271.
First unequivocal description in humans that foam cells are derived from monocyte-macrophages rather than smooth muscle cells, based on reactions in atheromatous plaques to monoclonal antibodies.

11.   ROSS R: **Platelet-derived growth factor.** *Annu Rev Med* 1987, 38:71–79.
Detailed and up-to-date review of PDGF and its role in atherogenesis.

12.   STEINBERG D: **Lipoproteins and the pathogenesis of atherosclerosis.** *Circulation* 1987, 76:508–514.
Plausible account of the role of oxidative modification of LDL as a mechanism for foam cell formation.

13.   MITCHINSON MJ, BALL RY, CARPENTER KLH, PARUMS DV: **Macrophages and ceroid in atherosclerosis.** In *Hyperlipidaemia and Atherosclerosis* edited by Suckling KE, Groot PHE. London: Academic Press, 1988, pp 117–134.
Detailed account of the origins of ceroid and its presence in atheromatous plaques, which provides support for the oxidized LDL hypothesis of foam cell formation.

14.   WISSLER RW: **Current status of regression studies.** In *Atherosclerosis Reviews 3* edited by Paoletti R, Gotto AM. New York: Raven Press, 1978, pp 213–229.

Review of data concerning regression of atherosclerosis, mainly confined to experimental animals.

15. ARMSTRONG ML, HEISTAD DA, MARCUS ML, PIEGORS DJ, ABOUD FM: **Haemodynamic sequelae of regression of experimental atherosclerosis.** *J Clin Invest* 1983, 71:104–113.
Sobering description of persisting functional abnormality in regressed vessels in experimental atherosclerosis, despite anatomical improvement.

16. JAGANNATHAN SN, CONNOR WE, BAKER WH, BHATTACHARYYA AK: **The turnover of cholesterol in human atherosclerotic arteries.** *J Clin Invest* 1974, 54:366–377.
Measurement of specific activity of cholesterol in several tissues including the arterial wall at varying intervals after injection of ^{14}C-cholesterol into patients with atherosclerosis.

17. SMALL DM, BOND MG, WAUGH D, PRACK M, SAWYER JK: **Physicochemical and histological changes in the arterial wall of non-human primates during progression and regression of atherosclerosis.** *J Clin Invest* 1984, 73:1590–1605.
Careful analysis of the physico-chemical changes occurring in experimentally induced atherosclerosis in non-human primates during regression.

18. MALINOW MR: **Regression of atherosclerosis in humans: fact or myth?** *Circulation* 1981, 64:1–3.
Review of pre-CLAS trial evidence that human atherosclerosis can sometimes regress.

19. BROWN BG, BOLSON EL, DODGE HT: **Arteriographic assessment of coronary atherosclerosis. Review of current methods, their limitations, and clinical applications.** *Arteriosclerosis* 1982, 2:2–15.
Description of the advantages of computer-assisted analysis versus visual assessment of coronary angiograms and data on the variations observed in lesion diameter on serial angiography.

20. LEVY RI, BRENSIKE JF, EPSTEIN SE, KELSEY SF, PASSAMANI ER, RICHARDSON JM, LOH IK, STONE NJ, ALDRICH RF, BATTAGLINI JW, MORIARTY DJ, FISHER ML, FRIEDMAN L, FRIEDEWALD W, DETRE KM: **The influence of changes in lipid values induced by cholestyramine and diet on progression of coronary artery disease: results of the NHLBI Type II Coronary Intervention Study.** *Circulation* 1984, 69:325–337.
Analysis of the results of the type II intervention trial which showed that prolonged therapy with cholestyramine helps prevent angiographic progression of coronary lesions but does not induce regression.

21. BLANKENHORN DH, NESSIM SA, JOHNSON RL, SANMARCO ME, AZEN SP, CASHIN-HEMPHILL L: **Beneficial effects of combined colestipol-niacin therapy on coronary atherosclerosis and coronary venous bypass grafts.** *JAMA* 1987, 257:3233–3240.
Well controlled demonstration that diet plus lipid-lowering drug therapy induced regression in 16% of lesions of coronary arteries and bypass grafts versus the 2% achieved by diet alone.

6

7 PRIMARY HYPERTRIGLYCERIDAEMIA

7

Introduction

Under this heading will be considered patients presenting with predominant hypertriglyceridaemia due to increases in fasting plasma of chylomicrons or VLDL or both (types I, IV or V phenotypes) but without any obvious secondary cause. Evidence of the hereditary basis of these disorders is often only presumptive but detailed investigation of first-degree relatives sometimes reveals partial metabolic defects, suggestive of recessive inheritance.

Familial lipoprotein lipase deficiency

This rare disorder, also known as familial type I hyperlipoproteinaemia, is characterized by marked hypertriglyceridaemia and chylomicronaemia which usually presents in childhood. It is due to the inheritance of a recessive gene which results in deficiency of the extrahepatic enzyme lipoprotein lipase, the rate-limiting step in chylomicron clearance. This results in a failure of chylomicron hydrolysis and accumulation of chylomicrons in plasma. Decreased uptake of dietary triglyceride by the liver presumably decreases VLDL secretion since VLDL levels remain normal; however, IDL and LDL are both reduced. The condition is very rare and affects less than one in a million persons [1]. The main clinical features are recurrent episodes of abdominal pain, often resembling acute pancreatitis, eruptive xanthomata and hepatosplenomegaly associated with serum triglycerides in the region of 50–100 mmol/l [2]. The accumulation of chylomicrons in plasma results in the appearance of lipaemia retinalis on ophthalmoscopy (Fig. 7.1).

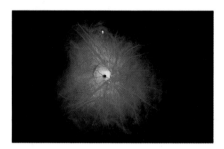

Fig. 7.1. Retinal photograph of patient with type I hyperlipoproteinaemia showing lipaemia retinalis.

7

The gross chylomicronaemia (see Fig. 4.1) results in an increase in serum cholesterol as well as triglyceride, but the plasma triglyceride : cholesterol mass ratio often exceeds 9 : 1. VLDL levels are usually normal or decreased, whereas LDL and HDL levels are both markedly reduced. The diagnosis depends upon demonstrating that plasma lipoprotein lipase levels, following an intravenous dose of heparin 5000 i.u., are less than 10% of normal. Measurement of PHLA can be misleading since plasma levels of hepatic lipase, phospholipase and monoglyceride lipase often rise normally after heparin administration. Lipoprotein lipase can be distinguished from these other enzymes by various techniques including inhibition by sodium chloride, protamine sulphate or specific antibodies, or by chromatographic separation on heparin-sepharose affinity columns (see Chapter 2). Some first-degree relatives exhibit 50% reductions in plasma or adipose tissue lipoprotein lipase, indicative of heterozygosity for the mutant gene.

The main line of treatment is to minimize chylomicron formation by decreasing the intake of long-chain triglyceride to less than 50 g/day. There appears to be no increased susceptibility to atherosclerosis in this condition, the chief complication being acute pancreatitis. Diagnosis of the latter is sometimes confused by the fact that hyperlipaemia interferes with the assay of serum amylase, giving rise to apparently normal levels despite clinical signs of acute pancreatitis. However, diluting serum up to 10-fold reveals an elevated serum amylase and confirms the diagnosis [3]. The risk of this occurring is minimized if plasma triglyceride levels can be kept below 20 mmol/l.

Familial lipoprotein lipase inhibitor

Type I hyperlipoproteinaemia has been ascribed to the presence of a circulating inhibitor of lipoprotein lipase in three generations of a single family. This resulted in marked chylomicronaemia and hypertriglyceridaemia in affected individuals, including a serum triglyceride of 27 mmol/l in a 4-month-old baby [4]. The disorder is characterized by absence of plasma PHLA despite increased levels of lipoprotein lipase in adipose tissue. Also, the lipoprotein-free fraction of patients' plasma inhibited the PHLA of normal plasma, indicating the presence of an inhibitor. The precise nature of the latter has not been established.

Familial apoC-II deficiency

This disorder is due to recessively inherited mutant genes which, in the homozygous state, result in the absence from plasma of normal apoC-II, with a consequent defect of lipolysis and hypertriglyceridaemia [5]. At least four distinct functionally inactive apoC-II variants have been described to date. Lipoprotein lipase is present in normal amounts but cannot hydrolyse chylomicrons or VLDL in the absence of normal apoC-II, which activates the enzyme in plasma. Addition of apoC-II *in vitro* restores to normal the PHLA in patients' plasma and the latter is inactive as a substrate for lipoprotein lipase unless apoC-II is added. The diagnosis can sometimes be made by demonstrating an absent or anomalous band of apoC-II on isoelectric focusing of delipidated VLDL. Heterozygotes exhibit a 30–50% decrease in apoC-II levels but remain normolipaemic.

Homozygotes have triglycerides in the range 15–107 mmol/l, with either a type I or type V phenotype, and often develop acute pancreatitis [6]. Premature vascular disease is unusual but has been described. The hypertriglyceridaemia responds dramatically to infusion of plasma from a normal subject, albeit only temporarily (Fig. 7.2). Similar results were obtained after injecting a synthetically prepared fragment of the biologically active portion of apoC-II into two apoC-II-deficient siblings [7].

7

Familial hepatic lipase deficiency

In 1974 a subject with hypertriglyceridaemia was described as having a novel form of dyslipoproteinaemia; this was termed hyperαtriglyceridaemia because of the accumulation of triglyceride in the HDL or α-lipoprotein fraction. Subsequently it was shown that both this Swedish patient and his brother had

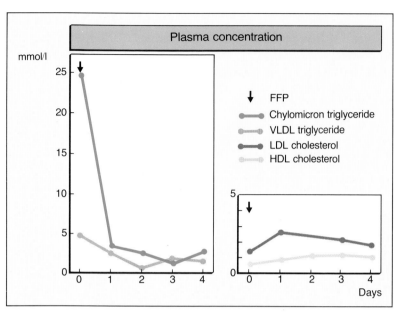

Fig. 7.2. Effects of intravenous infusion of 200 ml of fresh-frozen plasma (FFP) on plasma lipids in a patient with apoC-II deficiency. Adapted by permission from Miller *et al., Eur J Clin Invest* 1981, 11:69–76.

virtually no post-heparin hepatic lipase activity in plasma, whereas lipoprotein lipase activity was normal [8]. In the meantime, two Canadian brothers with this syndrome had been described [9]. The index patient had raised levels of both serum cholesterol and triglyceride, the latter ranging from 4.5 to 93 mmol/l depending upon diet. Corneal arcus, eruptive xanthomata and palmar striae were present together with evidence of myocardial ischaemia. His hyperlipidaemia failed to respond to clofibrate, despite the presence of β-VLDL and a type III pattern on lipoprotein electrophoresis.

Studies of the lipoprotein abnormalities present in hepatic lipase deficiency have revealed two characteristic features that lend support to the putative mode of action of this enzyme. Firstly, the HDL fraction consists solely of abnormally large, triglyceride-rich particles with the density of HDL_2, while HDL_3 particles are absent. This abnormality presumably reflects the lack of hydrolysis of HDL_2 triglycerides by hepatic lipase which normally leads to formation of HDL_3 from HDL_2. The second characteristic lipoprotein alteration is the accumulation of β-VLDL and IDL and the concomitantly raised ratio of cholesterol to triglycerides in VLDL [8,9]. Whereas lipoprotein lipase hydrolyses VLDL triglycerides, hepatic lipase has been postulated to attack VLDL remnants (β-VLDL and IDL). Therefore, deficiency of hepatic lipase should lead to the accumulation of VLDL remnants in blood, as indeed was the case in the Canadian and Swedish brothers with this condition. Since accumulation of cholesterol-rich VLDL remnants is the hallmark of type III hyperlipopro-teinaemia, which usually results from homozygosity for apoE$_2$, it is important to note that in both the Canadian and the Swedish hepatic lipase-deficient patients the apoE$_3$ isoform was present. Lipoprotein turnover studies in the Swedish index patient showed considerably decreased catabolism of small VLDL and IDL, while that of large VLDL was normal [10].

Of interest and importance for the clinical management of hepatic lipase de-ficiency is the pronounced difference between the Canadian and Swedish index patients. While the Canadian was grossly obese the Swede was slim. The Canadian not only had the phenotypic characteristics of type III hyper-lipoproteinaemia, but also signs and symptoms of ischaemic heart disease. The slender Swede had none of these abnormalities and is now aged 66 and in good health.

Familial hypertriglyceridaemia

Introduction

This disorder is usually subdivided according to whether the predominant phenotype of affected individuals is type IV or type V. However, there is sometimes overlap within families and it is probable that similar genetic ab-normalities are responsible for both varieties of the disorder but with a more severe expression in those with a type V phenotype.

7

Type IV

Familial type IV hyperlipoproteinaemia is characterized by moderate hypertri-glyceridaemia due to increased levels of VLDL. Goldstein *et al.* [11] studied the relatives of 23 hypertriglyceridaemic survivors of myocardial infarction and found a bimodal distribution of fasting triglycerides but a normal distri-bution of cholesterol values, consistent with an autosomal dominant pattern of inheritance. They estimated the frequency of the disorder in the population at 0.2–0.3% but noted that it was expressed less frequently than expected in childhood. Mean fasting values of serum cholesterol and triglyceride were 6.2 and 3.0 mmol/l, respectively, in their series of patients. The majority exhib-ited a type IV phenotype but some families also had members with a type V phenotype. In contrast with familial combined hyperlipidaemia (Chapter 9) none of the families contained individuals with type IIa or IIb phenotypes.

The nature of the genetic defect remains to be determined but affected subjects have larger than normal VLDL particles with an increased triglyc-eride:apoB ratio, accompanied by a decrease in HDL cholesterol [12]. Turnover studies show that VLDL triglyceride synthesis is increased to a greater extent than VLDL-apoB synthesis and that the fractional catabolic rate of both VLDL components is reduced [13,14]. The latter phenomenon appears to reflect saturation of a normal clearance mechanism in most instances rather than an intrinsic catabolic defect in that PHLA is usually normal. However, decreased uptake and re-esterification of fatty acid by adipose tissue has been reported [15], which could lead to accumulation of FFA and end-product inhibition of lipolysis despite normal enzyme levels. FFA flux into triglyceride is increased in type IV subjects, especially when they are placed on a high carbohydrate intake [16]. The increase in VLDL synthesis is accompanied by a decrease in the proportion of VLDL converted to LDL [17]. This, together with a reduction in cholesterol ester content of LDL, maintains plasma LDL cholesterol levels within the normal range, nor is there any increase in LDL-apoB levels, in contrast to familial combined hyperlipidaemia [12].

The underlying mechanism for the overproduction of VLDL triglyceride remains to be determined but affected members of type IV families have higher insulin levels than unaffected members, and show a positive correlation between plasma insulin and triglyceride (Fig. 7.3), suggesting that insulin resistance may be involved. The severity of hypertriglyceridaemia is aggravated by administration of corticosteroids or oestrogens, which can sometimes lead to acute pancreatitis. Glucose intolerance and hyperuricaemia are common accompaniments [18] but there are no specific clinical features or biochemical markers. There are conflicting data as to whether the risk of myocardial infarction is increased [11] or is not increased [19] above normal in this condition.

Management involves adherence to a modified fat diet designed to achieve ideal body weight, avoidance of sucrose and excess alcohol, and encouragement of physical activity. Should these methods fail, drug therapy may be required, either with nicotinic acid or with one of the fibrates. However, administration of the latter sometimes results in an undesirable rise in LDL, as is also observed when type IV patients are treated with the fish-oil preparation Maxepa [20].

Type V
This uncommon disorder has features of both type IV and type I hyperlipoproteinaemia, as would be expected in view of the increase in VLDL and chylomicrons which are its hallmark (see Fig 4.1). Unlike the type I disorder it seldom presents in childhood, and post-heparin lipoprotein lipase and hepatic lipase activities are usually normal. However, there is a similar liability to develop attacks of acute abdominal pain, which are often due to acute pancreatitis [1]. Other features are eruptive xanthomata, as shown in Fig. 7.4, glucose intolerance, hyperuricaemia and symptoms of peripheral neuropathy. The pancreatitis has been attributed to hydrolysis of triglyceride within the pancreas by lipase, the consequent release of FFA causing local damage to the gland. In some instances repeated attacks can result in chronic pancreatic insufficiency [21].

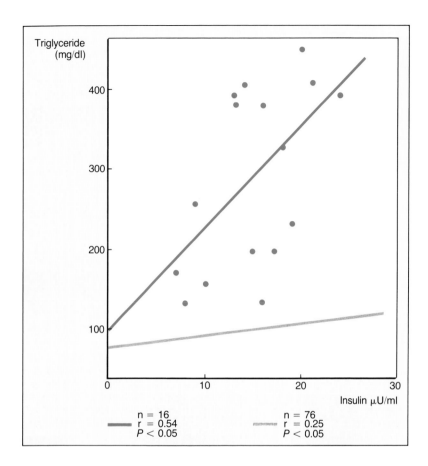

Fig. 7.3. Correlation between fasting plasma triglycerides and insulin levels in patients with familial hypertriglyceridaemia. Grey line represents best fit of data from normolipidaemic relatives. Adapted by permission from Brunzell and Bierman, *Ann Intern Med* 1977, 87:198–199.

Hypertriglyceridaemia in type V subjects is accentuated by obesity and alcohol consumption. There is a strong correlation between the triglyceride level and body weight but not all patients are obese [22]. The mode of inheritance is uncertain but, as mentioned previously, there seems to be a certain amount of overlap with familial type IV hyperlipoproteinaemia. In obese patients a type V phenotype will often change to a type IV pattern following successful introduction of a weight-reducing diet. Turnover studies show similar increases in VLDL apoB synthesis in type IV and V patients but a more marked decrease in fractional catabolic rate among the latter [17]. There is some evidence that

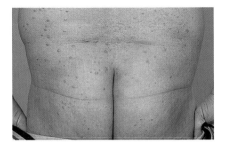

Fig. 7.4. Eruptive xanthomata in 33-year-old man with type V hyperlipoproteinaemia (fasting serum cholesterol 30, triglyceride 90 mmol/l, blood glucose 12 mmol/l, apoE phenotype E3/3).

the ε4 allele is unusually prevalent in type V hyperlipoproteinaemia but the significance of this association is obscure.

Although there have been isolated case reports of coronary disease in type V patients there was no evidence of undue predisposition to CHD in the 32 families studied by Greenberg et al. [22]. Acute pancreatitis is the major complication and every effort should be made to avoid precipitating factors such as oestrogens and alcohol so as to maintain triglyceride levels below 20 mmol/l. Dietary control is often difficult because administration of a low fat diet (< 50 g/day) to reduce chylomicronaemia sometimes increases VLDL synthesis. Lipolysis can be promoted by oxandrolone in males and norethindrone acetate in females [1] whereas triglyceride synthesis can be reduced by large doses of fish-oils rich in ω3 fatty acids, as discussed further in Chapter 12, or of nicotinic acid. The latter is especially useful in patients liable to repeated attacks by acute pancreatitis.

Annotated references

1.   NIKKILA EA: **Familial lipoprotein lipase deficiency and related disorders of chylomicron metabolism.** In *Metabolic Basis of Inherited Disease 5th edn* edited by Stanbury JB, Wyngaarden JB, Fredrickson DS, Goldstein JL, Brown MS. New York: McGraw Hill, 1983, pp 622–642.
An authoritative and comprehensive account of disorders of chylomicron clearance by that great Finnish lipidologist, the late Esko Nikkila.

2.   LEVY RI, RIFKIND BM: **Diagnosis and management of hyperlipoproteinemia in infants and children.** *Am J Cardiol* 1973, 31:547–556.
Short review of the diagnosis and therapy of the hyperlipoproteinaemias seen in childhood.

3.   FALLAT RW, VESTER JW, GLUECK CJ: **Suppression of amylase activity by hypertriglyceridemia.** *JAMA* 1973, 225:1331–1334.
First observation of the pitfall which may beset the laboratory diagnosis of an acute abdomen in association with chylomicronaemia.

4.   BRUNZELL JD, MILLER NE, ALAUPOVIC P, ST HILAIRE RJ, WANG CS, SARSON DL, BLOOM SR, LEWIS B: **Familial chylomicronemia due to a circulating inhibitor of lipoprotein lipase activity.** *J Lipid Res* 1983, 24:12–19.
Careful study of a unique family.

5.   BRECKENRIDGE WC, LITTLE A, STEINER G, CHOW A, POAPST M: **Hypertriglyceridemia associated with deficiency of apolipoprotein C-II.** *N Engl J Med* 1978, 298:1265–1273.
First description of a case of apoC-II deficiency, whose hypertriglyceridaemia dramatically improved after a blood transfusion.

6.   COX DW, BRECKENRIDGE WC, LITTLE JA: **Inheritance of apolipoprotein C-II deficiency with hypertriglyceridemia and pancreatitis.** *N Engl J Med* 1978, 299:1421–1427.
Description of seven cases of homozygous apoC-II deficiency, five of whom had experienced acute pancreatitis.

7.   BAGGIO G, MANZATO E, GABELLI C, FELLIN R, MARTINI S, ENZI GB, VERIATO F, BAIOCCHI MR, SPRECHER DL, KASHYAP ML, BREWER HB, CREPALDI G: **Apolipoprotein C-II deficiency syndrome. Clinical features, lipoprotein characterization, lipase activity, and correction of hypertriglyceridemia after apolipoprotein C-II administration in two affected patients.** *J Clin Invest* 1986, 77:520–527.
Demonstration of the beneficial effects of injecting synthetic apoC-II into two siblings who had inherited apoC-II$_{padua}$, an inactive variant.

8.   CARLSON LA, HOLMQUIST L, NILSSON-EHLE P: **Deficiency of hepatic lipase activity in post-heparin plasma in familial hyper-α-triglyceridaemia.** *Acta Med Scand* 1987, 219:435–447.
Detailed account of two Swedish brothers with familial deficiency of hepatic lipase.

9.   BRECKENRIDGE WC, LITTLE JA, ALAUPOVIC P, WANG CS, KUKSIS A, KAKIS G, LINDGREN F, GARDINER G: **Lipoprotein abnormalities associated with a familial deficiency of hepatic lipase.** *Atherosclerosis* 1982, 45:161–179.
Detailed account of clinical and laboratory features of two Canadian patients with inherited deficiency of hepatic lipase.

10.   DEMANT T, CARLSON LA, HOLMQUIST L, KARPE F, NILSSON-EHLE P, PACKARD CJ, SHEPHERD J: **Lipoprotein metabolism in hepatic lipase deficiency: studies on the turnover of apolipoprotein B and on the effect of hepatic lipase on high density lipoprotein.** *J Lipid Res* 1988, 29:1603–1611.
Turnover studies which demonstrate essential role of hepatic lipase in conversion of small VLDL and IDL to LDL.

11.   GOLDSTEIN JL, SCHROTT HG, HAZZARD WR, BIERMAN EL, MOTULSKY AG: **Hyperlipidemia in coronary heart disease. II. Genetic analysis of lipid levels in 176 families and delineation of a new inherited disorder, combined hyperlipidemia.** *J Clin Invest* 1973, 52:1544-1568.

7

This large study by Goldstein and colleagues helped establish the frequency of genetically determined forms of hyperlipidaemia in relation to CHD.

12. BRUNZELL JD, ALBERS JJ, CHAIT A, GRUNDY SM, GROSZEK E, MCDONALD GB: **Plasma lipoproteins in familial combined hyperlipidemia and monogenic familial hypertriglyceridemia.** *J Lipid Res* 1983, 24:147–155.

Comparison of differences in size and composition of VLDL, LDL and HDL particles in familial hypertriglyceridaemia and familial combined hyperlipidaemia.

13. CHAIT A, ALBERS JJ, BRUNZELL JD: **Very low density lipoprotein overproduction in genetic forms of hypertriglyceridaemia.** *Eur J Clin Invest* 1980, 10:17–22.

Comparison of the rates of turnover of VLDL-apoB and triglyceride in familial hypertriglyceridaemia and familial combined hyperlipidaemia.

14. KISSEBAH AH, ALFARSI S, ADAMS PW: **Integrated regulation of very low density lipoprotein triglyceride and apolipoprotein B kinetics in man: normolipemic subjects, familial hypertriglyceridemia and familial combined hyperlipidemia.** *Metabolism* 1981, 30:856–868.

Similar study to [11] but including data on percentage conversion of VLDL-apoB to LDL-apoB.

15. CARLSON LA, WALLDIUS G: **Fatty acid incorporation into human adipose tissue in hypertriglyceridaemia.** *Eur J Clin Invest* 1976, 6:195–211.

A study on a large population of normo- and hyperlipidaemic subjects demonstrating a decreased assimilation of fatty acids by adipose tissue *in vitro* in hypertriglyceridaemia.

16. QUARFORDT SH, FRANK A, SHAMES DM, BERMAN M, STEINBERG D: **Very low density lipoprotein triglyceride transport in type IV hyperlipoproteinaemia and the effects of carbohydrate-rich diets.** *J Clin Invest* 1970, 49:2281–2297.

A sophisticated analysis of the kinetics of triglyceride transport in normal and hypertriglyceridaemic subjects and the impact thereon of a high carbohydrate diet.

17. PACKARD CJ, SHEPHERD J, JOERNS S, GOTTO AM, TAUNTON OD: **Apolipoprotein B metabolism in normal, type IV and type V hyperlipoproteinemic subjects.** *Metabolism* 1980, 29:213–222.

Comparison of VLDL-apoB turnover in type IV and type V subjects analysed by the SAAM computer programme.

18. KWITEROVICH PO, MARGOLIS S: **Type IV hyperlipoproteinaemia.** *Clin Endocrinol Metab* 1973, 2:41–71.

Comprehensive account of the mechanisms of type IV hyperlipoproteinaemia including a detailed list of secondary causes.

19. BRUNZELL JD, SCHROTT HG, MOTULSKY AG, BIERMAN EL: **Myocardial infarction in the familial forms of hypertriglyceridemia.** *Metabolism* 1976, 25:313–320.

Analysis of families with familial hypertriglyceridaemia and familial combined hyperlipidaemia which shows increased frequency of myocardial infarction in the latter but not the former.

20.   SULLIVAN DR, SANDERS TAB, TRAYNER IM, THOMPSON GR: **Paradoxical elevation of LDL apoprotein B levels in hypertriglyceridaemic patients and normal subjects ingesting fish oil.** *Atherosclerosis* 1986, **61**:129–134.
First description that the triglyceride-lowering effect of fish-oil can lead to an undesirable rise in LDL-apoB.

21.   FALLAT RW, GLUECK CJ: **Familial and acquired type V hyperlipoproteinemia.** *Atherosclerosis* 1976, **23**:41–62.
Description of 29 adults with type V hyperlipoproteinaemia in 17 of whom this was considered to be familial, and of the accompanying pancreatitis.

22.   GREENBERG BH, BLACKWELDER WC, LEVY RI: **Primary type V hyperlipoproteinemia. A descriptive study in 32 families.** *Ann Intern Med* 1977, **87**:526–534.
Detailed account of familial type V hyperlipoproteinaemia which includes data on lipoprotein and hepatic lipase levels.

7

8 PRIMARY HYPERCHOLESTEROLAEMIA

<table>
<tr><td>

Introduction

Familial hypercholesterolaemia (FH)
Homozygous FH
Heterozygous FH
Laboratory diagnosis

Familial defective apoB$_{100}$

Polygenic hypercholesterolaemia

Familial hyperαlipoproteinaemia

Cholesterol ester storage disease

Annotated references

</td></tr>
</table>

8

Introduction

Primary hypercholesterolaemia includes all forms of predominant hyper-cholesterolaemia due to an increase in LDL or HDL for which there is no secondary cause. FH has an obvious genetic basis whereas evidence of this is less clear-cut in polygenic hypercholesterolaemia and familial hyperαlipoproteinaemia. Familial combined hyperlipidaemia, which some-times presents with hypercholesterolaemia alone, is dealt with in Chapter 9.

Familial hypercholesterolaemia (FH)

FH, also known as familial type II hyperlipoproteinaemia, affects approxi-mately 0.2% of the population. Commonly this is due to inheritance of one mutant gene encoding the LDL receptor which causes heterozygous FH. Very occasionally inheritance of two mutant genes occurs, giving rise to homozy-gous FH. Inheritance of two dissimilar mutants results in compound heterozygotes but these cannot be distinguished clinically from homozygotes and will be referred to as such [1].

The LDL receptor normally plays a major role in the catabolism of LDL and deficiency of LDL receptors results in accumulation of LDL in plasma as evidenced by hypercholesterolaemia from birth. Total cholesterol levels are roughly twice normal in adult heterozygotes and four times normal in homozygotes, as shown in Table 8.1. Triglyceride levels are usually normal in affected children, most of whom exhibit a type IIa phenotype, but a type IIb phenotype is quite common in adults. HDL cholesterol may be normal but is often reduced, especially in homozygotes.

Table 8.1. Range of plasma or serum cholesterol values observed in FH homozygotes and heterozygotes throughout the world.

Group	n	Total cholesterol (mmol/l)
Homozygotes	165	18.4–20.3
Heterozygotes	978	8.9–10.8

Data cited by Thompson et al. [10].

8

Four different classes of mutations of the LDL receptor which give rise to FH have been identified, each of which includes several distinct gene defects. As illustrated in Fig. 8.1, class 1 mutations represent null alleles which result in the complete absence of immunologically detectable receptors; class 2 alleles disrupt the transport to the cell surface of any receptors which are synthesized; class 3 alleles result in the formation of receptors which are functionally defective with respect to binding LDL; and class 4 alleles, the rarest, result in the formation of receptors which are normal in all respects except their inability to cluster in coated pits, which prevents them from being internalized after binding LDL [2]. So far 13 class 1 mutations have been identified, including one which occurs in over 60% of French-Canadians with FH, and involves a 10 kb deletion at the promotor end of the gene [3]. In addition, three class 2 mutations, two class 3 mutations, and five class 4 mutations have now been identified. Interestingly, all class 4 mutations have been shown to affect the cytoplasmic domain of the LDL receptor.

Homozygous FH

Clinically, homozygous FH is characterized by extreme hypercholesterolaemia and the onset in childhood of cutaneous xanthomata, which typically are planar (Fig. 8.2) or tuberose, plus tendon xanthomata and corneal arcus. Levels of cholesterol in plasma correlate inversely with the severity of the LDL receptor deficit, which depends upon the nature of the underlying gene defect [4]. The deficit is more marked with class 1 and 2 mutations

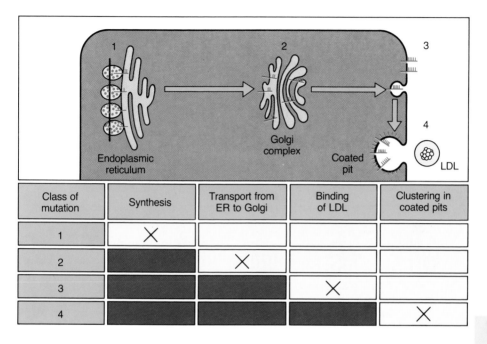

Class of mutation	Synthesis	Transport from ER to Golgi	Binding of LDL	Clustering in coated pits
1	X			
2	■	X		
3	■	■	X	
4	■	■	■	X

Fig. 8.1. Four classes of mutations at the LDL receptor locus. These mutations disrupt synthesis, transport, binding, and clustering of the LDL receptor in the cell. ER, endoplasmic reticulum. Adapted by permission from Goldstein and Brown, *J Lipid Res* 1984, 25:1450.

where there is an inability to produce receptors (receptor-negative) than with class 3 and 4 mutations when mature but abnormal receptors are formed (receptor-defective). Turnover studies show an almost complete absence of receptor-mediated catabolism of apoB, with a low fractional catabolic rate of both IDL and LDL. ApoB synthesis is twice normal, the increase being partly via a VLDL-independent pathway and imputed to direct secretion of LDL, and partly due to increased conversion of IDL to LDL (Fig. 8.3).

Atheromatous involvement of the aortic root is always evident by puberty as manifested by an aortic systolic murmur, a gradient across the aortic valve and angiographic narrowing of the aortic root together with coronary ostial stenosis [5]. Sudden death from acute coronary insufficiency before 30 was the rule before the recent introduction of better methods of treatment. At postmortem examination the aortic valve, sinuses of Valsalva and ascending arch

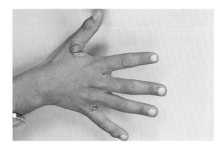

Fig. 8.2. Planar xanthomata in 12-year-old boy with homozygous FH.

8

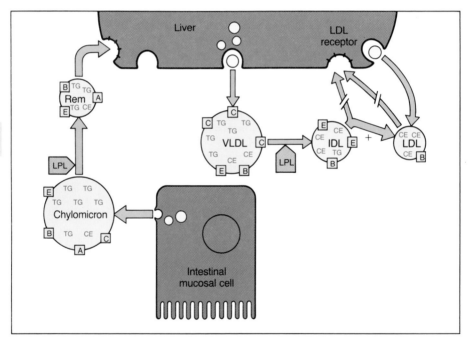

Fig. 8.3. Schematic diagram of the mechanisms responsible for increases in both IDL and LDL levels in familial hypercholesterolaemia. These comprise impaired uptake and catabolism of both IDL and LDL, together with increased conversion of IDL to LDL and direct synthesis of the latter.

of the aorta are grossly infiltrated with atheroma (Fig. 8.4), with similar but less severe changes in all other major arteries. The histology shows numerous foam cells and cholesterol crystals but is otherwise typical of atherosclerosis [6].

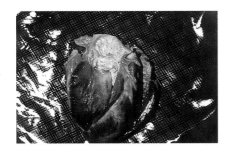

Fig. 8.4. Heart of male homozygote who died suddenly at 23, showing extensive atheroma of aortic root.

The chief determinant of the age of onset of CHD and the likelihood of premature death appears to be LDL receptor status [1]. Pooled data show that 60% of receptor-negative homozygotes exhibited CHD before the age of 10 years whereas this was never observed in receptor-defective patients until after that age. Furthermore, 26% of receptor-negative subjects had died from CHD before the age of 25 years compared with only 4% of receptor-defective homozygotes. Female gender does not protect against the cardiovascular complications of homozygous FH, in contrast to its prominent role in this respect in heterozygotes [7], possibly reflecting the lack in homozygotes of any sex difference in HDL cholesterol [8].

The management of homozygous FH presents a major therapeutic challenge. Dietary and drug regimens have little impact and the safest and most reliable means of reducing cholesterol levels is to undertake plasma exchange or LDL apheresis at 2-weekly intervals. Liver transplantation remedies the hepatic deficiency of LDL receptors and results in near-normal cholesterol levels but is hazardous and necessitates long-term immunosuppression. Although these measures slow the rate of progression of aorto-coronary atherosclerosis it may still be necessary to undertake coronary artery bypass grafting for coronary ostial stenosis and replace the aortic valve if this becomes significantly fibrosed.

Heterozygous FH

Nowadays screening the children or siblings of an affected subject should lead to early detection of heterozygous FH but all too often it remains undiagnosed until the onset of cardiovascular symptoms in adult life. In addition to hypercholesterolaemia there are often visible signs of cholesterol deposition, such as corneal arcus, xanthelasma and tendon xanthomata. Characteristic sites for the latter are the extensor tendons on the back of the hands and elbows, the Achilles tendons and the patellar tendon insertion into the pretibial tuberosity (Figs 8.5–8.8).

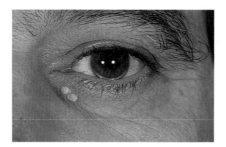

Fig. 8.5. Corneal arcus and xanthelasma in 47-year-old man with heterozygous FH.

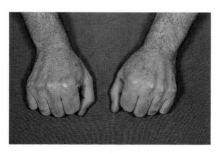

8

Fig. 8.6. Tendon xanthomata in extensor tendons of hands of patient shown in Fig. 8.5.

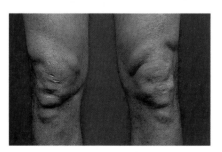

Fig. 8.7. Enlargement of pre-tibial tuberosities of patient shown in Fig. 8.5.

Tendon xanthomata, the clinical hallmark of FH, are an age-related phenomenon. Thus only 7% of heterozygotes below the age of 19 years exhibited tendon xanthomata in one series whereas these lesions were present in 75% of their parents [9]. This is further illustrated by an analysis of patients with definite heterozygous FH, i.e. hypercholesterolaemia plus tendon xanthomata in the patient or in a first-degree relative, attending 10 lipid clinics in Britain [10], as shown in Fig. 8.9. Mean pretreatment values of serum cholesterol

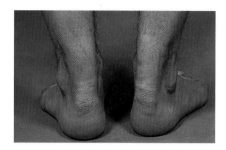

Fig. 8.8. Achilles tendon xanthomata of patient shown in Fig. 8.5.

were identical in patients of both sexes (10.4 mmol/l) despite the greater age of the females (40 versus 35 years). Overall the percentage of males and females with tendon xanthomata was very similar (75 and 72%, respectively) despite the higher HDL cholesterol of female heterozygotes, as observed by others [7]. However, a history of CHD was present in a higher proportion of males than females between the ages of 30 and 59, as shown in Fig. 8.10.

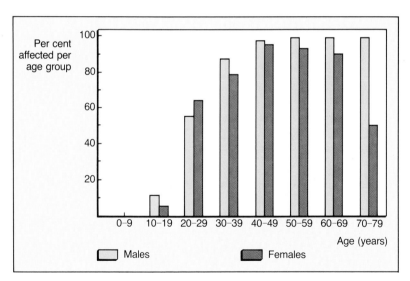

Fig. 8.9. Proportion of male and female heterozygotes with tendon xanthomata according to deciles of age. Adapted by permission of the American Heart Association [10].

The high frequency and premature onset of CHD in heterozygous FH has been well documented, as has its much lower incidence in females compared

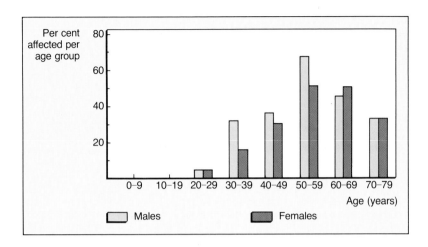

Fig. 8.10. Proportion of male and female heterozygotes with coronary heart disease (angina and/or history of myocardial infarction) according to deciles of age. Adapted by permission of the American Heart Association [10].

8

with males, in whom the onset of symptoms occurs 9–10 years earlier [11]. Females lose this advantage if they are smokers. If left untreated, up to 50% of males develop CHD by the age of 50 and, on angiography, over 70% of these have triple-vessel disease, including 32% with disease of the left main stem [12]. It has been estimated that CHD occurs about 20 years earlier in FH than in the remainder of the population, with a corresponding decrease in life expectancy if left untreated.

In one large series [7], no cases of CHD were observed in patients without tendon xanthomata. However, in subjects with tendon xanthomata, neither total nor LDL cholesterol differed between those with and without CHD. An inverse correlation between HDL cholesterol and CHD has been observed in patients of both sexes [13]. Male heterozygotes with a type IIb phenotype have lower HDL cholesterol values than those with a type IIa pattern, reflecting an inverse correlation between HDL cholesterol and plasma triglyceride, and their frequency of myocardial infarction is higher [14]. Recent data suggest that Lp(a) levels are much higher in FH heterozygotes with CHD than in those without, despite similar levels of LDL cholesterol (Seed *et al.*, unpublished data).

The influence of age, sex and lipid levels on the presence of tendon xanthomata and CHD is summarized in Table 8.2. An LDL cholesterol above 7.8 mmol/l seems to be a prerequisite for the development of both tendon xanthomata and CHD before the age of 50 years and the latter seldom occurs in the absence of tendon xanthomata. There is a strong association between being male and developing CHD, which is presumably related to the lower HDL cholesterol and higher triglyceride levels of men compared with women with FH. The absence of any relationship between HDL cholesterol and tendon xanthomata is noteworthy, implying as it does that cholesterol deposition and removal from extravascular tissues are unaffected by variations in plasma HDL which appear to influence CHD.

Table 8.2. Factors associated with development of tendon xanthomata and coronary heart disease in heterozygotes by age of 50 years.

	Tendon xanthomata	Coronary heart disease
Increasing age	+ +	+ +
Male sex	−	+ +
Increased LDL-cholesterol*	+	+
Decreased HDL-cholesterol	−	+
Increased triglyceride	−	±
Tendon xanthomata		±

*> 7.8 mmol/l. Published by permission from Thompson, *J Inher Metab Dis* 1988, 11 (suppl 1):18–28 and Kluwer Academic Publishers.

Turnover studies show a roughly 50% decrease in receptor-mediated catabolism of LDL-apoB which results in a reduced fractional catabolic rate and prolonged half-life of LDL in plasma. LDL-apoB synthesis is often increased but all these abnormalities are less marked than in homozygotes. The cholesterol : apoB ratio of LDL is raised, reflecting a relative increase in the proportion of light LDL present in plasma [15].

8

The treatment of heterozygous FH usually involves drug therapy with an anion-exchange resin such as cholestyramine. In adult patients with a type IIb phenotype this may need supplementing with nicotinic acid or one of the fibric acid derivatives. Combination drug therapy is often necessary to achieve optimal control of hypercholesterolaemia and elimination of other risk factors is vital, especially smoking. Partial ileal bypass is occasionally useful in patients who are intolerant of resins. The effectiveness of all these approaches is markedly enhanced by concomitant administration of an HMG CoA reductase inhibitor, such as lovastatin. The recent advent of LDL apheresis, which selectively removes LDL but not HDL, holds promise, especially when used in conjunction with an HMG CoA reductase inhibitor. Despite these measures it is sometimes necessary to resort to coronary artery bypass grafting, especially in those with left main stem disease. Postoperative control of hypercholesterolaemia is crucial if graft atherosclerosis is to be avoided.

Laboratory diagnosis

Often the diagnosis of FH is obvious, as when tendon xanthomata are found in a hypercholesterolaemic subject. However, the diagnosis is less straightforward in children and in adults lacking this pathognomonic sign.

As discussed elsewhere [15], antenatal diagnosis of homozygous FH can be undertaken by culturing fetal cells from amniotic fluid and showing them by binding studies to have less than 5% of the normal complement of LDL receptors. A similar approach can be undertaken later in life using cultured skin fibroblasts, although this is tedious and time-consuming.

Diagnosis of heterozygous FH at birth is best achieved by measuring LDL cholesterol in cord blood. It has been shown that most infants with a cord blood LDL cholesterol of > 1.06 mmol/l have an LDL cholesterol above the 95th centile after the age of 1 year but measuring total cholesterol in cord blood is unhelpful. Between the ages of 1 and 16 years, serum total cholesterol levels are nearly twice as high in heterozygotes as in their unaffected siblings but the diagnosis cannot be made with confidence when the value is in the range 6.5–7.0 mmol/l, even in children known to have an affected parent. Detection of FH by measuring serum total cholesterol in the population at large is even more problematical, due to a high proportion of false positives in children with normal LDL levels and of false negatives in children with FH. This emphasizes the need to determine LDL cholesterol rather than total cholesterol when screening for FH in childhood, the 95th centile values of LDL cholesterol between the ages of 6 and 15 averaging 3.3 mmol/l in males and 3.5 mmol/l in females.

Cuthbert et al. [16] recently described a functional assay of LDL receptors on lymphocytes cultured in lipoprotein-deficient serum in the presence of lovastatin, based upon the greater amount of LDL required by FH cells to respond to stimulation with phytohaemagglutinin. However, there have been problems in getting this assay to work in other laboratories, which suggests that it does not quite meet the pressing need for a reliable biochemical test for FH.

Familial defective apoB$_{100}$

Using gene probes it has been recently shown that a single base substitution in the codon for arginine 3500 in the apoB gene gives rise to a form of apoB$_{100}$ which impairs the ability of LDL to bind to the LDL receptor [17]. Affected individuals have moderate hypercholesterolaemia without any hallmarks other than a raised LDL. IDL appears to be cleared normally, in contrast to FH, presumably via binding of its apoE to the LDL receptor. In view of the size of the gene there seems a strong likelihood that other mutations affecting the receptor-binding domain of apoB$_{100}$ may also exist and could represent a hitherto unrecognized cause of monogenic hypercholesterolaemia within families.

Polygenic hypercholesterolaemia

Plasma cholesterol levels are under the control of many different genes and environmental factors the summated effects of which result in a near-Gaussian distribution of cholesterol levels in the population. Clustering in an individual of several genes which tend to induce moderate elevations of plasma cholesterol should theoretically result in polygenic hypercholesterolaemia. Indeed, Goldstein *et al*, in their study of survivors of myocardial infarction (see ref. [9] in Chapter 9), identified a group of patients with elevated plasma cholesterol levels which had no evidence of bimodality of cholesterol concentrations in the families of affected probands. Instead the distribution of cholesterol in these families was unimodal but shifted towards a higher mean level. This entity was defined as polygenic hypercholesterolaemia and was attributed to several independent genes clustering in an individual. In patients with primary hypercholesterolaemia not due to FH the frequency of the ε4 allele is significantly increased. As discussed previously, this allele is associated with elevated LDL-cholesterol in the general population and may well be one of the genes contributing to polygenic hypercholesterolaemia [18].

The disorder can be delineated only by family studies. The classic clinical features of familial hypercholesterolaemia do not occur in polygenic hypercholesterolaemia but the disorder does appear to be associated with premature atherosclerosis. Estimates of the prevalence of polygenic hypercholesterolaemia will vary according to the arbitrary definition of the upper limit of normal for serum cholesterol. Goldstein *et al* identified it in 14% of their hyperlipidaemic survivors of myocardial infarction, using a value of 7.4 mmol/l as their cut-off, as compared with the 10% who had FH. Obviously the lower the cut-off value used, the higher is the estimated frequency of polygenic hypercholesterolaemia relative to FH in the population at large.

Familial hyperαlipoproteinaemia

Hyperαlipoproteinaemia, defined as an HDL cholesterol level above the 90th percentile, sometimes occurs on a familial basis. Familial hyperαlipoprotein-aemia is a heterogeneous entity in that some families show a clear-cut autosomal dominant pattern of inheritance while in others the features suggest interaction between polygenic influences and common environmental factors within the household. The increase in HDL cholesterol reflects rises in both HDL_2 and HDL_3 [19]. The syndrome tends to be associated with a decreased frequency of CHD and with longevity [20]. Affected individuals require reassurance rather than treatment.

In most instances the mechanism of familial hyperαlipoproteinaemia is unknown but a subgroup of patients has been described in whom the increase in HDL cholesterol is due to deficiency of cholesterol ester transfer activity in plasma. This results in smaller than normal LDL particles and enlarged HDL particles, rich in apoE. Such individuals may exhibit corneal opacities and can develop CHD [21].

Cholesterol ester storage disease

A rare cause of primary hypercholesterolaemia is inherited deficiency of cholesterol ester hydrolase, which gives rise to cholesterol ester storage disease. LDL cholesterol is increased whereas HDL cholesterol is reduced. Clinically the disorder is characterized by hepatic and splenic enlargement but xanthomata are absent. Diagnosis depends upon demonstrating excessive amounts of cholesterol ester in liver biopsies and deficiency of cholesterol ester hydrolase activity in cultured fibroblasts. Accelerated atherosclerosis has been described.

8

Annotated references

1.   GOLDSTEIN JL, BROWN MS: **Familial hypercholesterolemia**. In *The Metabolic Basis of Inherited Disease 5th edn* edited by Stanbury JB, Wyngaarden JB, Fredrickson DS, Goldstein JL, Brown MS. New York: McGraw-Hill, 1983, pp 672–712.
A classic monograph on the disease which led the authors to discover the LDL receptor and win the Nobel Prize.

2.   RUSSELL DW, LEHRMAN MA, SUDHOF TC, YAMAMOTO TC, DAVIS CG, HOBBS HH, BROWN MS, GOLDSTEIN JL: **The LDL receptor in familial hypercholesterolemia: use of human mutations to dissect a membrane protein**. *Cold Spring Harbor Symposia on Quantitative Biology* 1986, **51**:811–819.
Relatively recent review of the molecular genetics of familial hypercholesterolaemia.

3.   HOBBS HH, LEITERSDORF E, GOLDSTEIN JL, BROWN MS, RUSSELL DW: **Multiple crm⁻ mutations in familial hypercholesterolemia**. *J Clin Invest* 1988, **81**:909–917.
Description of the 13 mutations identified to date which result in a complete failure of LDL receptor synthesis.

4.   Sprecher DL, Hoeg JM, Schaefer EJ, Zech LA, Gregg RE, Lakatos E, Brewer HB Jr: **The association of LDL receptor activity, LDL cholesterol level, and clinical course in homozygous familial hypercholesterolaemia.** *Metabolism* 1985, 34:294–299.
Study of 13 homozygotes at NIH which shows inverse correlation between LDL receptor activity in fibroblasts and the biochemical and clinical severity of the disorder.

5.   Allen JM, Thompson GR, Myant NB, Steiner R, Oakley CM: **Cardiovascular complications of homozygous familial hypercholesterolaemia.** *Br Heart J* 1980, 44:361–368.
Description of the clinical and angiographic features of the cardiovascular complications of homozygous FH, as observed in seven patients.

6.   Buja LM, Kovanen PT, Bilheimer DW: **Cellular pathology of homozygous familial hypercholesterolemia.** *Am J Pathol* 1979, 97:327–345.
A post-mortem study of the morbid anatomy and histology of atheroma in four FH homozygotes.

7.   Gagné C, Moorjani S, Brun D, Toussaint M, Lupien P-J: **Heterozygous familial hypercholesterolemia. Relationship between plasma lipids, lipoproteins, clinical manifestations and ischaemic heart disease in men and women.** *Atherosclerosis* 1979, 34:13–24.
Large study of over 500 FH heterozygotes in Quebec which examines the relationship between serum lipid abnormalities and the presence of tendon xanthomata and coronary disease.

8.   Seftel HC, Baker SG, Sandler MP, Forman MB, Joffe BI, Mendelsohn D, Jenkins T, Mieny CJ: **A host of hypercholesterolaemic homozygotes in South Africa.** *Br Med J* 1980, 281:633–636.
The high prevalence of FH in the Transvaal enabled the authors to describe the clinical course of 34 homozygotes and their variable susceptibility to increases in LDL.

9.   Kwiterovich PO, Fredrickson DS, Levy RI: **Familial hypercholesterolaemia (one form of familial type II hyperlipoproteinaemia).** *J Clin Invest* 1974, 53:1237–1249.
Very detailed analysis of distribution of cholesterol levels in over 200 children born of 90 heterozygote-normal matings.

10.   Thompson GR, Seed M, Niththyananthan, McCarthy S, Thorogood M: **Genotypic and phenotypic variation in familial hypercholesterolaemia.** *Arteriosclerosis* 1989, 9 (suppl):I75–I80.
Analysis of some of the factors responsible for inter- and intrafamilial variations in the phenotypic expression of FH, including apoE phenotype.

11.   Slack J: **Risk of ischaemic heart disease in familial hyperlipoproteinaemic states.** *Lancet* 1969, ii:1380–1382.
The first study to document the greatly increased risk of coronary heart disease in heterozygous FH.

12.   Sugrue DD, Thompson GR, Oakley CM, Trayner IM, Steiner RE: **Contrasting patterns of coronary atherosclerosis in normocholesterolaemic smokers and patients with familial hypercholesterolaemia.** *Br Med J* 1981, 283:1358–1360.

8

Angiographic description of differences in the pattern and severity of coronary disease in FH heterozygotes and normocholesterolaemic smokers.

13.   STREJA D, STEINER D, KWITEROVICH PO: **Plasma high density lipoproteins and ischemic heart disease: studies in a large kindred with familial hypercholesterolemia.** *Ann Intern Med* 1978, **89**:871–880.
Study of a large family which first demonstrated the inverse correlation between HDL cholesterol and coronary heart disease in FH.

14.   MOORJANI S, GAGNÉ C, LUPIEN P-J, BRUN D: **Plasma triglycerides related decrease in high density lipoprotein cholesterol and its association with myocardial infarction in heterozygous familial hypercholesterolemia.** *Metabolism* 1986, **35**:311–316.
Analysis of the association between raised triglycerides, low HDL cholesterol and increased frequency of MI in FH heterozygotes.

15.   THOMPSON GR: **The hyperlipidaemias.** In *Genetic and Metabolic Disease in Pediatrics* edited by Lloyd JK, Scriver CR. London: Butterworths, 1985, pp 211–233.
Description of the major forms of hyperlipidaemia seen in childhood.

16.   CUTHBERT JA, EAST CA, BILHEIMER DW, LIPSKY PE: **Detection of familial hypercholesterolemia by assaying functional low density lipoprotein receptors on lymphocytes.** *N Engl J Med* 1986, **314**:879–883.
Ingenious but tricky assay of LDL receptor activity in lymphocytes designed to help diagnose FH.

17.   MCCARTHY BJ, SORIA L, LUDWIG EM, INNERARITY TL, GRUNDY SM, VEGA GL, MAHLEY RW, WEISGRABER KH: **An arginine 3500 glutamine mutation in familial defective apoB-100 subjects with LDL defective in binding to the apoB$_1$E (LDL) receptor.** *Circulation* 1988, **78** (suppl II):II66.
First description of the apoB gene defect responsible for impaired binding of LDL to its receptor, a novel cause of monogenic hypercholesterolaemia.

18.   UTERMANN G: **Apolipoprotein polymorphism and multifactorial hyperlipidaemia.** *J Inher Metab Dis* 1988, **11** (suppl I):74–86.
Review article by an author who has pioneered much of the work on apolipoprotein polymorphism.

19.   ISELIUS L, LALOUEL JM: **Complex segregation analysis of hyperalphalipoproteinemia.** *Metabolism* 1982, **31**:521–523.
Re-appraisal of the original family study of hyperalipoproteinaemia carried out by Glueck and colleagues (see [20]).

20.   GLUECK CJ, FALLAT RW, MILLETT F, GARTSIDE P, ELSTON RC, GO RCP: **Familial hyper-alpha-lipoproteinemia: studies in eighteen kindreds.** *Metabolism* 1975, **24**:1243–1265.
Description of the possible mode of inheritance of hyperalipoproteinaemia in 18 families, within which a history of longevity was common.

8

21. YAMASHITA S, MATSUZAWA Y, OKAZAKI M, KAKO H, YASUGI T, AKIOKA H, HIRANO K, TARUI S: **Small polydisperse low density lipoproteins in familial hyperalphalipo-proteinemia with complete deficiency of cholesteryl ester transfer activity.** *Atherosclerosis* 1988, 70:7–12.

Description of lipoprotein abnormalities observed in patients with hyperαlipoproteinaemia due to primary cholesterol ester transfer deficiency.

8

9 PRIMARY MIXED HYPERLIPIDAEMIAS

Introduction

Type III hyperlipoproteinaemia

Familial combined hyperlipidaemia

Hyperapoβlipoproteinaemia

Familial LCAT deficiency

Fish-eye disease

Annotated references

Introduction

This heading covers a disparate group of disorders with little in common other than the presence of a mixed form of hyperlipidaemia. In some instances hypertriglyceridaemia and hypercholesterolaemia are equally prominent, as in type III hyperlipoproteinaemia, whereas in others the increase is predominantly in cholesterol, as often occurs in familial combined hyperlipidaemia, or mainly in triglyceride, as is usual in LCAT deficiency and fish-eye disease. In the latter disorders hypertriglyceridaemia is often mild but is accompanied by marked decreases in HDL cholesterol.

Type III hyperlipoproteinaemia

This disorder, also known as familial dysβlipoproteinaemia [1], is characterized by the accumulation in plasma of chylomicron and VLDL remnants which fail to get cleared at a normal rate by hepatic receptors. *In vitro* the LDL or apoB,E receptor binds with high-affinity particles containing either $apoE_3$ or $apoE_4$; the latter differs from $apoE_3$ in the substitution of arginine for cysteine at position 112 in the amino acid sequence. However, particles containing $apoE_2$, in which there is substitution of cysteine for arginine at position 158, show virtually no binding to the apoB,E receptor [2]. Most patients with type III hyperlipoproteinaemia are homozygous for this form of $apoE_2$ but some are heterozygous, with $apoE_2/E_3$ or $apoE_2/E_4$ phenotypes [3]. In addition type III hyperlipoproteinaemia has been reported in association with the rare variants of $apoE_2$ and $apoE_3$ listed in Table 9.1, each of which exhibits reduced binding to the LDL receptor as compared with normal $apoE_3$. The disorder has also been described in individuals with complete deficiency of apoE [4].

Table 9.1. Some of the apolipoprotein E polymorphisms associated with type III hyperlipoproteinaemia.

Name	Charge relative to parent E3	Molecular defect	Receptor binding activity relative to E3
E1-Harrisburg[†]	−2	$Lys_{146} \rightarrow$ Glu	Defective
E3-A[‡]	0	$Cys_{112} \rightarrow$ Arg, $Arg_{142} \rightarrow$ Cys	<5%
E3-Leiden	0	Tandem repeat of residues 121–127[§]	25%
E2	−1	$Arg_{158} \rightarrow$ Cys	<2%
E2*	−1	$Arg_{145} \rightarrow$ Cys	45%
E2**	−1	$Lys_{146} \rightarrow$ Gln	40%
E2-Christchurch	−1	$Arg_{136} \rightarrow$ Ser	41%
E-Bethesda	−2	—	—
E-Deficiency	—	—	—

[†]Rall et al., J Clin Invest 1989, 83:1095–1011; [‡]Mann et al., Arteriosclerosis 1988, 8:612a; [§]Wardell et al., personal communication. Adapted by permission from Wardell et al., J Clin Invest 1987, 80:483–490. © American Society for Clinical Investigation.

9

Inheritance of a defective form of apoE is usually insufficient *per se*, however, to give rise to clinically evident type III hyperlipoproteinaemia in that the frequency of the $apoE_2/E_2$ phenotype in most populations is $1:100$ whereas the prevalence of this form of hyperlipidaemia is only $1:5000$. It seems that in addition to inheritance of a defective form of apoE other metabolic abnormalities must also be present before hyperlipidaemia will ensue. These include obesity, diabetes, hypothyroidism or other genetic disorders such as FH and familial combined hyperlipidaemia [5]. These presumably compound the remnant clearance defect either by decreasing apoB,E receptor expression, as occurs in FH and hypothyroidism, or by increasing VLDL synthesis and thus promoting remnant formation, as occurs in obesity and familial combined hyperlipidaemia. Similarly, a high fat intake promotes chylomicron remnant formation. The various mechanisms which contribute to the genesis of type III hyperlipidaemia are illustrated in Fig. 9.1.

Hormonal influences are also important in that type III hyperlipoproteinaemia seldom presents in males before puberty and in females it is rare before

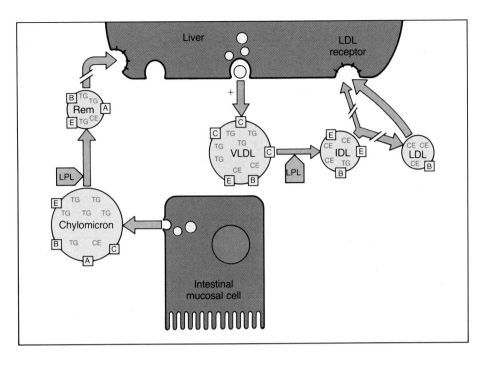

Fig. 9.1. Defective uptake of chylomicron remnants and IDL by the liver, with reduced conversion of IDL to LDL, is the primary metabolic abnormality in type III hyperlipoproteinaemia but this is compounded by secondary factors such as increased synthesis of chylomicrons or VLDL.

9

the menopause. Clinical features include corneal arcus, xanthelasma, tuberoeruptive xanthomata and, pathognomonically, palmar striae (Fig. 9.2). Typical sites for xanthomata are the knees and elbows (Fig. 9.3). Serum cholesterol and triglyceride are both elevated, usually to about 10 mmol/l, and lipoprotein electrophoresis shows the 'broad β' band characteristic of remnant particles. On ultracentrifugation the d < 1.006 fraction contains cholesterol-rich remnants which have β-mobility on lipoprotein electrophoresis (β-VLDL); a mass ratio of cholesterol : triglyceride of > 0.42 in this fraction is considered pathognomonic of the type III disorder, with the rare exception of hepatic lipase deficiency. The diagnosis should be confirmed by apoE phenotyping whenever possible (see Chapter 4). LDL cholesterol is reduced because of decreased conversion of IDL to LDL [2]. Despite this, atherosclerosis is common and presumably reflects the atherogenic properties of the β-VLDL particles, which are avidly taken up by macrophages. Histologically, however, the lesions are unremarkable [6]. Vascular disease occurs in over 50% of patients, involving not only the coronary tree but also peripheral and cerebral vessels.

Glucose intolerance and hyperuricaemia are also common. Acute pancreatitis can sometimes occur.

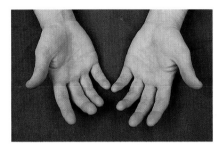

Fig. 9.2. Yellowish palmar striae in 35-year-old man with type III hyperlipoproteinaemia. Serum cholesterol 19, triglyceride 12 mmol/l, apoE$_2$/E$_2$.

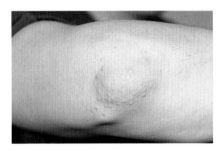

Fig. 9.3 Tubero-eruptive xanthomata on elbow of patient described in Fig. 9.2.

9

Management of type III hyperlipoproteinaemia involves remedying any obvious precipitating factors, such as hypothyroidism, diabetes, obesity or iatrogenic influences (Fig. 9.4). In addition, most patients will require therapy with a fibric acid derivative such as bezafibrate or gemfibrozil. Providing body weight can be controlled by diet, administration of one of these drugs, either alone or together with nicotinic acid, usually results in virtual normalization of serum lipids, rapid regression of cutaneous xanthomata and amelioration of ischaemic symptoms. Anion-exchange resins aggravate the hypertriglyceridaemia and should be avoided [7]. HMG CoA reductase inhibitors are sometimes useful, especially in double heterozygotes for type III and FH [8].

Familial combined hyperlipidaemia

This entity was first described in 1973 by Goldstein *et al.* [9] on the basis of detailed family studies of hyperlipidaemic patients who survived a myocardial infarction. They showed that 30% of such individuals manifested el-

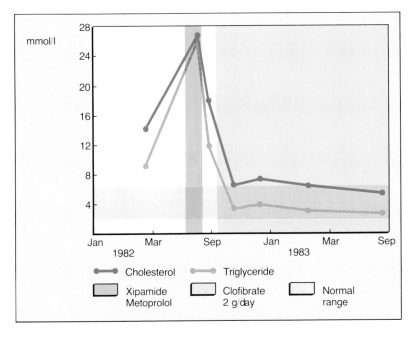

Fig. 9.4. Aggravation of hyperlipidaemia in a hypertensive patient with type III hyperlipoproteinaemia by a beta blocker and a thiazide diuretic and its partial amelioration when these drugs were withdrawn. Subsequent administration of a fibric acid derivative resulted in near-normalization of serum lipids. Adapted by permission from Thompson, *Br J Clin Pract* 1987, 41:47–51.

9

evations of both cholesterol and triglyceride, with a variable pattern of phenotypic expression within families. Overall roughly 50% of the relatives of affected subjects are hyperlipidaemic, of whom one-third have hypercholesterolaemia (type IIa), one-third have hypertriglyceridaemia (type IV or V) and one-third have both abnormalities (type IIb). Goldstein *et al.* concluded that the disorder was inherited in a monogenic manner but other authors have claimed that the pattern of transmission is more consistent with polygenic inheritance [10]. This issue cannot be resolved until a distinct biochemical marker becomes available. Whatever the mode of inheritance the disorder is undoubtedly familial and relatively common, occurring in up to 0.5% of the general population. Familial combined hyperlipidaemia (FCH) differs from FH in that affected children never show a type IIa phenotype, hypertriglyceridaemia being the earliest manifestation of the disorder, and it differs from familial hypertriglyceridaemia in that the latter is never associated with type IIa or IIb phenotypes.

The nature of the genetic defect is unknown but the disorder is characterized by increased synthesis of $apoB_{100}$, as manifested by high rates of turnover of both VLDL and LDL-apoB [11]. VLDL-triglyceride synthesis is also increased but to a lesser extent than in familial hypertriglyceridaemia whereas VLDL-apoB synthesis is increased to a more marked extent than in the latter disorder [12]. Furthermore, the proportion of VLDL particles converted to LDL is normal in FCH whereas it is subnormal in familial hypertriglyceridaemia [13]. ApoB levels are raised in FCH, usually reflecting increases in LDL but sometimes reflecting increases in VLDL-apoB [14]. VLDL particle size tends to be reduced, in contrast to familial hypertriglyceridaemia, and the concentration of IDL is increased. The LDL cholesterol:apoB ratio and HDL cholesterol concentration both tend to be on the low side, especially in subjects with marked hypertriglyceridaemia.

There are no distinctive clinical features in FCH and the diagnosis depends upon demonstrating multiple phenotypes within the family. However, such studies are not easily performed in a routine clinical setting and individuals with a type IIb phenotype who do not have tendon xanthomata or any secondary cause are often regarded as presumptive cases of FCH.

The condition is undoubtedly associated with an increased risk of atherosclerosis and it is estimated that it occurs in at least 15% of patients with CHD below the age of 60 [11]. In contrast with familial hypertriglyceridaemia there is a definite increase in the risk of myocardial infarction in FCH, as illustrated in Table 9.2.

9

Table 9.2 Myocardial infarction in living relatives.	
Familial combined hyperlipidaemia (24 families)	
Hyperlipidaemic relatives	10/57 (17.5%)
Normolipidaemic relatives	5/94 (5.3%)
Familial hypertriglyceridaemia (19 families)	
Hyperlipidaemic relatives	2/43 (4.7%)
Normolipidaemic relatives	2/61 (3.3%)
Data from Brunzell *et al.*, *Metabolism* 1976, 25:313–320.	

Diet alone is often insufficient to control FCH. The main aim of therapy is to reduce excessive synthesis of VLDL and one way of achieving this is by administration of nicotinic acid. Fibric acid derivatives are easier to take but have the drawback in type IV patients of promoting conversion of VLDL to LDL and thereby increasing LDL cholesterol. This problem can be overcome by concomitant administration of either an anion-exchange resin or an HMG CoA reductase inhibitor. The combination of gemfibrozil and lovastatin seems to be a particularly effective means of controlling hypertriglyceridaemia, reducing LDL cholesterol and raising HDL cholesterol in FCH [15]. However, because of the possibility of myopathy, combined therapy with fibrates and HMG CoA reductase inhibitors should be used with caution.

Hyperapoβlipoproteinaemia

The term 'hyperapoβlipoproteinaemia' (hyperapoB) was first coined by Sniderman et al. [16] to describe a syndrome characterized by an increased concentration of LDL-apoB (> 120 mg/dl) in plasma despite a normal concentration of LDL cholesterol (< 5 mmol/l). Affected individuals are often hypertriglyceridaemic, and show an apparent predisposition to clinically manifest atherosclerosis of the coronary, cerebral and peripheral arteries. These features are also found in FCH and there is considerable overlap between the two entities. An increase in VLDL-apoB synthesis is seen in both disorders, as illustrated in Fig. 9.5, which leads to an increased rate of formation and thus an expanded pool of LDL-apoB, despite LDL being catabolized at a normal rate [17]. This occurs without a corresponding increase in LDL-cholesterol because the major subfraction of LDL, 'heavy' LDL, has a subnormal cholesterol : protein ratio in hyperapoB subjects, especially those with hypertriglyceridaemia [18]. The probable mechanism is increased exchange of cholesteryl ester for triglyceride between 'light' LDL, the precursor of 'heavy' LDL, and VLDL; this results in the formation of 'heavy' LDL which is depleted in cholesteryl ester relative to its protein content. In normal subjects 'heavy' LDL has a cholesterol : apoB ratio of 1.33, whereas in hypertriglyceridaemic hyperapoB subjects the corresponding value is 0.88, the particles being smaller and denser than normal.

Since hyperapoB exhibits similar phenotypic features to FCH and both disorders seem to have the same metabolic defect, namely overproduction of apoB, this suggests that they may be identical. However, FCH is considered to be a dominantly inherited disorder, whereas the pattern of distribution of hyperapoB within families is compatible with polygenic inheritance. Until such time as the genetic defect or defects responsible have been identified it seems reasonable to keep an open mind as to whether primary hypoapoB represents a subgroup of FCH patients with type IV phenotypes or a genetically distinct disorder.

There are no special clinical features although an association between raised LDL-apoB levels and xanthelasma has been reported [19], an example of which is shown in Fig. 9.6. Tendon xanthomata occurred in members of two families with hyperapoB and phytosterolaemia but were not found in hyperapoB relatives without phytosterolaemia [20]. However, we have observed them in an hyperapoB patient without sitosterolaemia and they have also been reported in association with an elevated VLDL-apoB [21]. It is important to exclude other possible causes of tendon xanthomata in normocholesterolaemic individuals, such as β-sitosterolaemia and cerebro-tendinous xanthomatosis [22].

9

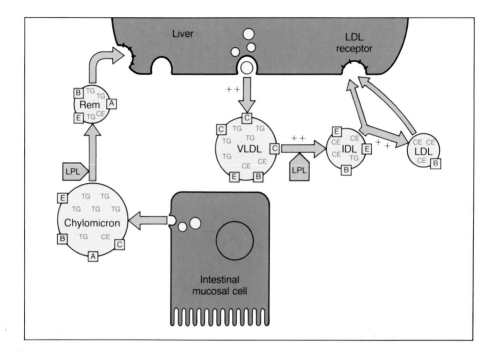

9

Fig. 9.5. Increased synthesis of LDL-apoB secondary to increased synthesis of VLDL-apoB with normal apoB catabolism characterize familial combined hyperlipidaemia and hyperapoβlipoproteinaemia.

Familial LCAT deficiency

Familial deficiency of LCAT is a rare disorder characterized clinically by diffuse corneal opacities (see Fig. 9.7), haemolytic anaemia, proteinuria, and hypertriglyceridaemia. It was first described in 1967 in a Norwegian family by Norum and Gjone and subsequently a further 26 families with a total of 50 affected homozygotes have been found [23]. The chief consequence of deficiency of LCAT is an inability to esterify free cholesterol in plasma, which results in the accumulation in all lipoprotein fractions of free cholesterol and lecithin, together with a decrease in lysolecithin (see Chapter 2). The increase in free cholesterol also occurs in erythrocytes and results in target cells and a normochromic anaemia.

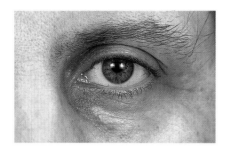

Fig. 9.6. Xanthelasma in type IV patient with hyperapoβlipoproteinaemia. Total cholesterol 6.9, triglyceride 3.3 mmol/l and LDL-apoB 151 mg/dl.

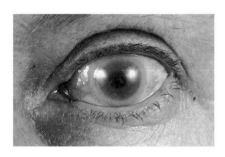

Fig. 9.7. Corneal opacification in female with familial LCAT deficiency. Published by permission from Borysiewicz *et al.*, *Q J Med* 1982, 51:411–426.

Serum cholesterol is often normal but HDL cholesterol is greatly decreased, as is the percentage of esterified cholesterol present in plasma (< 20% versus > 66% normally). The only cholesterol esters present in plasma are those formed by intestinal ACAT. Fasting triglycerides are usually moderately elevated, reflecting increases in VLDL as well as the presence of abnormal, triglyceride-rich LDL particles. Three different-sized subfractions of LDL can be identified and the largest of these has been incriminated in the renal failure which frequently complicates this disorder and is characterized by extensive lipid deposition in the kidneys. A similar process is presumably involved in the genesis of the corneal opacities although the deficiency of HDL may also play a role, by impairing reverse cholesterol transport. The HDL particles that are present resemble nascent HDL, showing a 'stacked-disc' appearance on electron microscopy and becoming spherical if exposed to LCAT.

Lipoprotein electrophoresis shows virtual absence of HDL and Lp-X is present on agar gel electrophoresis (see Fig. 3.4). Confirmation of the diagnosis depends upon demonstrating absence of LCAT activity in plasma and its partial deficiency in heterozygous relatives, in whom the disorder is otherwise silent. The gene for LCAT has now been cloned and the heterogeneous expression of the disorder between families suggests that several different mutations will eventually be identified. So far gene analysis has not revealed any major deletions or rearrangements of DNA in LCAT-deficient individuals but point mutations have not been excluded. Ideally, treatment should consist in injecting patients with biosynthetically prepared LCAT but this is not yet available. Transfusions of fresh plasma cause temporary improvement but are not really practicable on a long-term basis. Other measures involve placing patients on a low-fat diet in an attempt to minimize the concentration of the large molecular weight LDL particles which are thought to be involved in causing renal failure. The latter has necessitated long-term dialysis or renal transplantation in several instances and is the major life-threatening complication of LCAT deficiency.

Fish-eye disease

Fish-eye disease was first described in 1979 by Carlson and Philipson and altogether only three cases have been reported, all Swedish [23]. The disorder is named after the characteristic corneal opacities which are similar to but much more marked than those in familial LCAT deficiency and which, unlike the latter, cause visual impairment. Although it has a familial tendency the disorder differs from LCAT deficiency in the lack of anaemia and renal damage.

Fasting triglycerides were moderately elevated because of increases in VLDL and IDL but cholesterol levels were within the normal range. The percentage of cholesterol esters in whole plasma was slightly reduced but the most striking change was a marked reduction in HDL, reflecting major decreases in both apoA-I and cholesterol ester content. LCAT activity was normal when the patient's own lipoproteins were used as substrate but only 10–15% of normal when an exogenous substrate was used. These findings led Carlson and Holmquist to suggest that there are two forms of LCAT activity in plasma, one which acts only on HDL (α-LCAT) and one which acts on VLDL and LDL (β-LCAT). They further demonstrated that fish-eye disease is due to deficiency of α-LCAT alone whereas familial LCAT deficiency is due to deficiency of both activities [24]. Assuming that only one gene is defective in LCAT deficiency this explanation implies that fish-eye disease results from a failure of a post-translational step which normally is responsible for conversion of β-LCAT into α-LCAT.

Annotated references

1.   HAVEL RJ: Familial dysbetalipoproteinemia. New aspects of pathogenesis and diagnosis. *Med Clin N Am* 1982, 66:441–454.

Useful and authoritative monograph on type III hyperlipoproteinaemia.

2.   MAHLEY RW, INNERARITY TL, RALL SC, WEISGRABER KH: **Plasma lipoproteins: apolipo-protein structure and function.** *J Lipid Res* 1984, 25:1277–1294.
Good review article on structure–function relationships of apolipoproteins with particular emphasis on role of abnormal apoE isoforms in type III hyperlipoproteinaemia.

3.   BRESLOW JL, ZANNIS VI, SANGIACOMO TR, THIRD JLHC, TRACY T, GLUECK CJ: **Studies of familial type III hyperlipoproteinemia using as a genetic marker the apoE phenotype E2/E2.** *J Lipid Res* 1982, 23:1224–1235.
Description of two out of 17 type III patients shown to be heterozygous for apoE$_2$.

4.   SCHAEFER EJ, GREGG RE, GHISELLI G, FORTE TM, ORDOVAS JM, ZECH LA, BREWER HB JR: **Familial apolipoprotein E deficiency.** *J Clin Invest* 1986, 78:1206–1219.
Clinical and biochemical features of apoE deficiency.

5.   BROWN MS, GOLDSTEIN JL, FREDRICKSON DS: **Familial type 3 hyperlipoproteinemia (dysbetalipoproteinemia).** In *The Metabolic Basis of Inherited Disease 5th edn* edited by Stanbury JB, Wyngaarden JB, Fredrickson DS, Goldstein JL, Brown MS. New York: McGraw Hill, 1983, pp 655–671.
Comprehensive account of the prevalence, presentation and pathogenesis of type III hyper-lipoproteinaemia.

6.   CABIN HC, SCHWARTZ DE, VIRMANI R, BREWER HB, ROBERTS WC: **Type III hyperlipo-proteinemia: quantification, distribution, and nature of atherosclerotic coronary arterial narrowing in five necropsy patients.** *Am Heart J* 1981, 102:830–835.
Description of the similarity between the histology of coronary lesions in patients with types II, III and IV hyperlipidaemia.

7.   MORGANROTH J, LEVY RI, FREDRICKSON DS: **The biochemical, clinical and genetic features of type III hyperlipoproteinemia.** *Ann Intern Med* 1975, 82:158–174.
A pre-apoE account of the physical signs and vascular complications of 49 type III patients seen at the National Institutes of Health.

8.   THOMPSON GR, FORD J, JENKINSON M, TRAYNER I: **Efficacy of mevinolin as adjuvant therapy for refractory familial hypercholesterolaemia.** *Q J Med* 1986, 60:801–809.
Early description of the usefulness of lovastatin (mevinolin) in the management of severe hyperlipidaemia.

9.   GOLDSTEIN JL, SCHROTT HG, HAZZARD WR, BIERMAN EL, MOTULSKY AG: **Hyperlipi-demia in coronary heart disease. II. Genetic analysis of lipid levels in 176 fam-ilies and delineation of a new inherited disorder, combined hyperlipidemia.** *J Clin Invest* 1973, 52:1544–1568.
First description of familial combined hyperlipidaemia and evidence that it is monogenically inherited, based on analysis of the relatives of hypercholesterolaemic and hypertriglyceri-daemic survivors of myocardial infarction in Seattle.

10.   NIKKILA EA, ARO A: **Family study of serum lipids and lipoproteins in coronary heart disease.** *Lancet* 1973, i:954–959.

9

Similar findings to those of Goldstein *et al.* [9] but a different interpretation in that the Finnish authors concluded that multiple-type or combined hyperlipidaemia was polygenically determined.

11.   GRUNDY SM, CHAIT A, BRUNZELL JD: **Familial combined hyperlipidaemia workshop.** *Arteriosclerosis* 1987, 7:203–207.

Brief review of current opinions on the definition, causation, prevalence and treatment of familial combined hyperlipidaemia.

12.   CHAIT A, ALBERS JJ, BRUNZELL JD: **Very low density lipoprotein overproduction in genetic forms of hypertriglyceridaemia.** *Eur J Clin Invest* 1980, 10:17–22.

See Chapter 7, reference [11].

13.   KISSEBAH AH, ALFARSI S, ADAMS PW: **Integrated regulation of very low density lipoprotein triglyceride and apolipoprotein B kinetics in man: normolipemic subjects, familial hypertriglyceridemia and familial combined hyperlipidemia.** *Metabolism* 1981, 30:856–868.

See Chapter 7, reference [12].

14.   BRUNZELL JD, ALBERS JJ, CHAIT A, GRUNDY SM, GROSZEK E, MCDONALD GB: **Plasma lipoproteins in familial combined hyperlipidemia and monogenic familial hypertriglyceridemia.** *J Lipid Res* 1983, 24:147–155.

See Chapter 7, reference [10].

15.   EAST C, BILHEIMER DW, GRUNDY SM: **Combination drug therapy for familial combined hyperlipidemia.** *Ann Intern Med* 1988, 109:25–32.

Comparison of efficacy of gemfibrozil alone versus gemfibrozil combined with colestipol or lovastatin in the treatment of type IIb and type IV patients with FCH.

16.   SNIDERMAN A, SHAPIRO S, MARPOLE D, SKINNER B, TENG B, KWITEROVICH PO: **Association of coronary atherosclerosis with hyperapobetalipoproteinemia [increased protein but normal cholesterol levels in human low density (t) lipoproteins].** *Proc Natl Acad Sci USA* 1980, 77:604–608.

First description of hyperapoβlipoproteinaemia, as observed in normocholesterolaemic patients with coronary disease.

17.   TENG B, SNIDERMAN AD, SOUTAR AK, THOMPSON GR: **Metabolic basis of hyperapobetalipoproteinemia. Turnover of apolipoprotein B in low density lipoprotein and its precursors and subfractions compared with normal and familial hypercholesterolemia.** *J Clin Invest* 1986, 77:663–672.

Detailed kinetic analysis of apoB turnover in hyperapoβlipoproteinaemia compared with FH.

18.   TENG B, THOMPSON GR, SNIDERMAN AD, FORTE FM, KRAUSS RM, KWITEROVICH PO: **Composition and distribution of low density lipoprotein fractions in hyperapobetalipoproteinemia, normolipidemia and familial hypercholesterolemia.** *Proc Natl Acad Sci USA* 1983, 80:6662–6666.

Description of density gradient ultracentrifugation of LDL into two major subfractions, 'light' and 'heavy' LDL, and their composition in normal subjects and various forms of hyperlipidaemia.

9

19.   DAVIGNON J, SING CF, LUSSIER-CACAN S, BOUTHILLIER D: **Xanthelasma, latent dyslipo-proteinemia and atherosclerosis: contribution of apoE polymorphism.** In *Latent Dyslipoproteinemias and Atherosclerosis* edited by de Gennes JL, Polonovski J, Paoletti R. New York: Raven Press, 1984, pp 213–223.
Observation that patients with normolipidaemic xanthelasma have higher LDL-apoB levels than control subjects.

20.   KWITEROVICH PO, BACHORIK PS, SMITH H, MCKUSICK VA, CONNOR WE, TENG B, SNIDERMAN AD: **Hyperapobetalipoproteinaemia in two families with xanthomas and phytosterolaemia.** *Lancet* 1981, i:466–469.
Perplexing study of Amish families showing co-existence of phytosterolaemia, tendon xanthomata and hyperapoβlipoproteinaemia in some members ('homozygotes') and hyperapoβlipoproteinaemia alone in others ('heterozygotes').

21.   VEGA GL, ILLINGWORTH DR, GRUNDY SM, LINDGREN FT, CONNOR WE: **Normo-cholesterolemic tendon xanthomatosis with overproduction of apolipoprotein B.** *Metabolism* 1983, 32:118–125.
Description of type IV patient with tendon xanthomata which were attributed to increased turnover of apoB despite normal concentration of LDL-apoB in plasma.

22.   MYANT NB: *The Biology of Cholesterol and Related Steroids.* London: Heinemann, 1981.
Classic reference work on sterol metabolism and disorders thereof.

23.   MCINTYRE N: **Familial LCAT deficiency and fish-eye disease.** *J Inher Metab Dis* 1988, 11 (suppl 1):45–56.
Short review article on the pathogenesis and clinical features of familial LCAT deficiency and fish-eye disease and the relationship between these two mainly Scandinavian disorders.

24.   CARLSON LA, HOLMQUIST L: **Evidence for deficiency of high density lipoprotein lecithin:cholesterol acyltransferase activity (α-LCAT) in fish eye disease.** *Acta Med Scand* 1985, 218:189–196.
Experiments showing inability of plasma from fish-eye disease patients to esterify free cholesterol in HDL despite normal esterification of cholesterol in VLDL and LDL.

9

10 SECONDARY HYPERLIPIDAEMIA

Introduction

Hormonal influences
Pregnancy
Exogenous sex-hormones
Hypothyroidism

Metabolic disorders
Diabetes mellitus — *juvenile onset, maturity onset*
Gout
Obesity
Progressive partial lipodystrophy
Storage disorders

Renal dysfunction
Nephrotic syndrome
Chronic renal failure, on dialysis or post-transplant

Obstructive liver disease

Toxins
Alcohol
Dioxin and chlorinated hydrocarbons

Iatrogenic
Antihypertensives
Immunosuppressants
Other drugs

Miscellaneous causes

Annotated references

10

Introduction

Hyperlipidaemia can be secondary to a number of diseases, hormonal disturbances and iatrogenic agents. Furthermore it can present with any of the phenotypes associated with primary hyperlipoproteinaemia and can have similar consequences. As with primary disorders the type II and IV phenotypes occur most often, especially type IV. A comprehensive account of secondary causes of the latter has been published by Kwiterovich and Margolis [1].

Although many of the disorders listed can cause hyperlipidaemia in their own right it is increasingly apparent that the most marked abnormalities tend to occur in those individuals who have a genetic susceptibility to environmental and constitutional influences.

Hormonal influences

Pregnancy
Pregnancy is normally accompanied by moderate increases in both cholesterol and triglyceride, which revert to normal *post partum.* These changes reflect increases in VLDL, LDL and HDL, due mainly to the increase in oestrogens. Marked rises in cholesterol are usual in FH but in one instance LDL cholesterol decreased quite markedly and tendon xanthomata regressed during pregnancy [2]. Pregnancy can markedly exacerbate hypertriglyceridaemia, especially where this is due to lipoprotein lipase deficiency.

Exogenous sex-hormones
The LRC Prevalence Study showed that women below the age of 45 on oral contraceptives had higher serum cholesterol and triglycerides than women not taking them. These differences reflected increases in VLDL and LDL but were not apparent in women over the age of 45 on oestrogen replacement therapy, who instead had higher HDL cholesterol levels than those of similar age not on oestrogens [3]. The taking of oestrogens is reported to be associated with a significant reduction in cardiovascular mortality in women in that age group and has been shown to decrease LDL levels in post-menopausal women with hypercholesterolaemia.

However, in some instances oestrogens, whether given as a contraceptive or replacement therapy, or for the treatment of prostatic cancer, cause marked hypertriglyceridaemia [4], severe enough to precipitate acute pancreatitis. The mechanism probably involves either an oestrogen-induced decrease in lipolysis or an increase in VLDL synthesis, due to enzyme-induction. The effect of the progestogenic component of the contraceptive pill varies according to whether this is norethisterone or levonorgestrel, both of which decrease HDL_2 cholesterol, or desogestrel, which does not.

Oral contraceptives are best avoided altogether by women at increased risk of CHD but modern low-dose oestrogen preparations containing a non-HDL-

10

lowering progestogen or the latter given alone are safer than older preparations with a high oestrogen content. Testosterone analogues, which increase hepatic lipase, have been used successfully in the past to treat type V hyperlipoproteinaemia in males, but administration of methyl testosterone to a genotypic female who had undergone a sex-change caused severe hyperlipidaemia and premature CHD [5]. Anabolic steroids cause marked decreases in HDL cholesterol.

Hypothyroidism
Hypothyroidism has long been recognized as an important and relatively common cause of reversible hyperlipidaemia. Usually this presents as hypercholesterolaemia with a type IIa or IIb phenotype but it can also manifest itself as a type III or IV phenotype. HDL cholesterol levels are sometimes elevated as well as LDL cholesterol. The increase in LDL is due to a decrease in receptor-mediated catabolism, similar to that seen in FH but reversible, as illustrated in Fig. 10.1.

A recent survey of over 2000 men and women in Scotland showed that 4% of those with a serum cholesterol > 8 mmol/l had unequivocal hypothyroidism and a further 8% had raised thyroid-stimulating hormone (TSH) levels suggestive of subclinical thyroid deficiency [6]. Most of these individuals were females and the data suggest that up to 20% of women over 40 with this degree of hypercholesterolaemia may be hypothyroid. The presence of an elevated TSH in such circumstances warrants a trial of L-thyroxine although this should be undertaken with due care in case it aggravates any associated myocardial ischaemia.

Screening those with less marked hypercholesterolaemia for hypothyroidism is unrewarding. However, hypothyroidism can precipitate type III hyperlipoproteinaemia in those with an ε2 allele and can accentuate the hypercholesterolaemia of FH. A T4 and TSH should be measured in all such patients, especially if their hyperlipidaemia is unresponsive to therapy.

10

Metabolic disorders

Diabetes mellitus
Juvenile onset
Untreated juvenile onset, type I or insulin-dependent diabetes mellitus (IDDM) is accompanied by ketosis and marked hypertriglyceridaemia, often with a type V phenotype. The latter is partly due to deficiency of lipoprotein lipase consequent on the lack of insulin and partly due to an increased flux of FFA from adipose tissue, which promotes hepatic triglyceride synthesis. FFA levels decrease, lipoprotein lipase levels rise and hypertriglyceridaemia

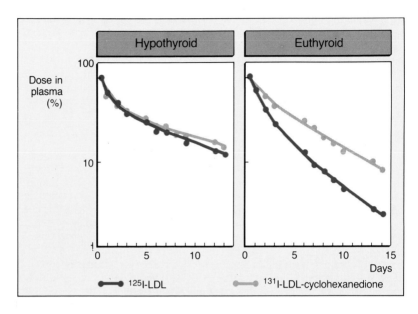

Fig. 10.1. Turnover of ^{125}I-LDL and ^{131}I-LDL-cyclohexanedione in a patient when hypothyroid (left) and euthyroid (right). The difference in the rates of turnover of the native and cyclohexanedione-coupled LDL after treatment with thyroxine indicates restoration to normal of receptor-mediated LDL catabolism. Adapted by permission from Thompson *et al., Proc Natl Acad Sci USA* 1981, 78:2591–2595.

10

rapidly comes under control with insulin replacement therapy [7]. The latter also reduces LDL levels if these are raised and increases HDL levels to normal or even above normal, compared with non-diabetic controls. However, goodness of control of diabetes as judged by haemoglobin A_1 HbA_1, seems to correlate better with blood glucose levels than with HDL cholesterol.

In contrast to macrovascular disease in poorly controlled IDDM, which is probably related to hyperlipidaemia, there is no difference in serum lipids between diabetics with and without proliferative retinopathy.

Maturity onset
Maturity onset, type II or non-insulin dependent diabetes mellitus (NIDDM) is more common than IDDM, usually comes on after the age of 40 and is often associated with obesity. It seems to be particularly common in Asians. Plasma insulin levels are normal or raised and the disorder is characterized by insulin resistance, that is to say a defect at the cellular level which impairs insulin-mediated disposal of glucose [7].

The commonest lipid abnormality is hypertriglyceridaemia, usually type IV, due mainly to increased synthesis of VLDL. This is the result of an increased input of substrates for triglyceride synthesis into the liver and leads to the production of large VLDL particles. Although clearance of triglyceride is probably impaired, due to decreased lipoprotein lipase activity, the proportion of VLDL converted to LDL is decreased and LDL levels are often normal. These features are illustrated in Fig. 10.2.

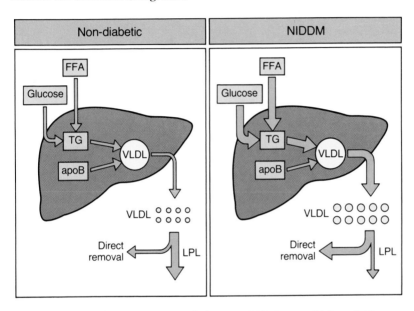

Fig. 10.2. Multiple changes in VLDL metabolism in NIDDM. Increased influx of FFA and glucose induce a disproportionate increase in triglyceride production, although apoB production may also be elevated, especially if subjects are obese. VLDL in plasma are increased in number and enriched in triglyceride, as indicated by the large circles. Clearance is decreased because of lower amounts of LPL, but there is more direct removal of VLDL. Adapted by permission [7].

10

Although the concentration of LDL cholesterol is often normal, its content of triglyceride tends to be higher than normal. Also, up to 5% of the lysine residues in apoB may be glycosylated, which decreases receptor-mediated uptake of LDL and promotes its deposition in the vessel wall.

HDL cholesterol is often reduced in NIDDM and may play a role in the pathogenesis of the atherosclerotic vascular disease which commonly occurs [8]. The hyperglycaemia and hypertriglyceridaemia respond well to a high-fibre, modified fat diet [9] or to sulphonyl ureas or insulin [10] but HDL total cholesterol does not change much. However, rate zonal density gradient ultracentrifugation shows that insulin therapy increases HDL_2 at the expense of HDL_3, presumably because it stimulates adipose tissue lipoprotein lipase activity, as illustrated in Fig. 10.3.

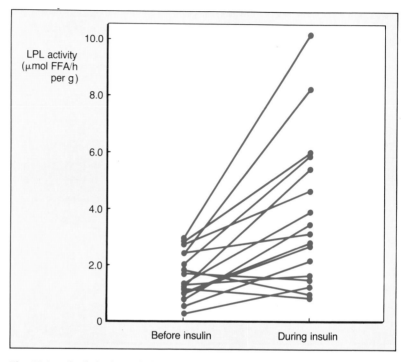

Fig. 10.3. Individual values of adipose tissue LPL activity before and during insulin therapy in non-insulin-dependent diabetics. Adapted by permission from Taskinen *et al.*, *Arteriosclerosis* 1988, 8:168–177.

10

The ability of fibrates to increase lipoprotein lipase activity, reduce plasma triglycerides, raise HDL cholesterol, and potentiate the action of hypoglycaemic agents, makes them appropriate treatment for diabetics whose hyperlipidaemia persists despite correction of hyperglycaemia. HMG CoA reductase inhibitors may also have a role to play in diabetics with persistent elevation of LDL cholesterol [11].

Gout

Hypertriglyceridaemia is a common accompaniment of gout. In one series eight out of 33 patients with primary hyperuricaemia and normal renal function had a fasting triglyceride of > 2 mmol/l, two of whom had values

> 14 mmol/l [12]. One of these had a type V phenotype, the remainder were type IV. There appears to be no direct metabolic link between hyperuricaemia and hypertriglyceridaemia, in that treatment with allopurinol has no effect on triglyceride levels, and the relationship may simply reflect the fact that obesity, alcohol and thiazides are common causes of both abnormalities. However, patients with primary type IV hyperlipoproteinaemia often have raised uric acid levels and it has been reported that some fibrates, notably fenofibrate, reduce both triglyceride and uric acid levels in such individuals. In contrast nicotinic acid compounds can reduce triglycerides but aggravate hyperuricaemia.

Obesity
Hypertriglyceridaemia, glucose intolerance, hyperinsulinism and vascular disease all commonly accompany obesity, which in these respects resembles maturity-onset diabetes. HDL cholesterol is also low, being inversely correlated with body weight, and rises with weight reduction [13]. Total cholesterol and LDL levels are often normal but turnover studies show increased rates of synthesis of both cholesterol and apoB. Although accompanied by an increase in the fractional catabolic rate of apoB this is insufficient to prevent an increase in pool size [14].

Progressive partial lipodystrophy
This rare disorder, which is sometimes familial, usually affects females and is characterized by the progressive loss of subcutaneous fat from the upper half of the body. Sometimes this is associated with apparent redistribution of fat, resulting in gross obesity of the lower limbs. Other features are glucose intolerance, which may progress to frank diabetes, hepatic dysfunction, severe hypertriglyceridaemia (type IV or V) and glomerulo-nephritis [15]. The cause of the disorder is unknown.

10

Storage disorders
Hypertriglyceridaemia is a feature of both Gaucher's disease and glycogen storage disease and has been shown to remit following creation of a portacaval shunt.

Renal dysfunction

Nephrotic syndrome
Hyperlipidaemia, often severe, is common in the nephrotic syndrome and was present in 17 out of 19 patients in a recent series [16]. Hypoalbu-

minaemia appears to play a central role probably by diverting increased amounts of FFA to the liver and thus stimulating lipoprotein synthesis. Other causes of hypoalbuminaemia can have the same effect. The commonest phenotypes are types IIa and IIb although type IV and V phenotypes can also occur. Serum cholesterol is inversely correlated with serum albumin (Fig. 10.4) and falls temporarily after albumin infusions. Accelerated vascular disease can be a major consequence of persistent hyperlipidaemia and was difficult to treat in the past, since fibrates frequently precipitated myositis. However, the advent of HMG CoA reductase inhibitors may offer a new hope to these patients.

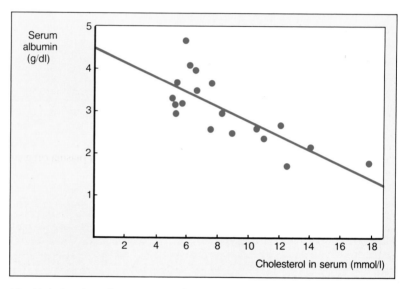

Fig. 10.4. Correlation between serum albumin and serum total cholesterol ($r = -0.78$, $P < 0.01$) in patients with the nephrotic syndrome. Adapted by permission [16].

10

Chronic renal failure, on dialysis or post-transplant

Hyperlipidaemia is common in patients with chronic renal failure, including those on haemodialysis, but in contrast to the nephrotic syndrome hypertriglyceridaemia, usually type IV, is much commoner than hypercholesterolaemia. This appears to be secondary to impaired lipolysis, possibly because of inhibition of lipoprotein lipase by an unknown factor present in uraemic plasma. Fibrates can restore lipoprotein lipase activity to normal in haemodialysed patients but must be used with caution because of the risk of myositis.

Patients undergoing haemodialysis have increased concentrations of remnant particles in plasma and decreased concentrations of HDL cholesterol, both of which presumably contribute to their increased risk of CHD [17]. Hyperlipidaemia also appears to be common in patients on chronic ambulatory peritoneal dialysis (CAPD), although the pattern differs from that seen with haemodialysis, possibly reflecting the absence of heparin administration in CAPD. Hyperlipidaemia often persists after successful renal transplantation although elevations in LDL as well as VLDL (type IIb) are commoner than in haemodialysed patients [18]. Immunosuppressive drugs probably play an important role in the genesis of post-transplant hyperlipidaemia, especially steroids.

Obstructive liver disease

Primary biliary cirrhosis or prolonged cholestasis from other causes is accompanied by marked hyperlipidaemia, due to the presence of high concentrations of Lp-X [19]. The latter is also found in familial LCAT deficiency but in biliary obstruction its presence reflects substrate excess rather than enzyme deficiency, due to the reflux of biliary lecithin into plasma. This interacts with free cholesterol, albumin and apoC in plasma and if these events occur at a rate which exceeds the cholesterol-esterifying capacity of LCAT, Lp-X is formed. Demonstration of the presence of Lp-X in jaundiced plasma on agar gel electrophoresis (see Fig. 3.4) is diagnostic.

Cutaneous xanthomata occur if hyperlipidaemia is marked (Fig. 10.5), sometimes accompanied by xanthomatous neuropathy but without accelerated atherosclerosis, as first pointed out by Ahrens and colleagues 40 years ago. Effective control of the hyperlipidaemia may require extreme measures such as plasma exchange, as discussed in Chapter 13. Fibrates can aggravate the hypercholesterolaemia whereas anion-exchange resins are ineffective. HMG CoA reductase inhibitors may cause myopathy in patients with cholestasis due to decreased biliary excretion.

10

Toxins

Alcohol
Ethanol is a common cause of secondary hypertriglyceridaemia, especially in males, and usually results in a type IV or V phenotype. Even moderate consumption of alcohol on a regular basis results in significantly higher serum triglycerides than are found in total abstainers. The hypertriglyceridaemic effect of alcohol is most marked in subjects with pre-existing primary type IV hyperlipoproteinaemia, and is enhanced by concomitant consumption of fat. One postulated mechanism is that ethanol is preferentially oxidized in the liver, which results in sparing of FFA and thus an increased availability of

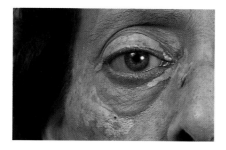

Fig. 10.5. Extensive xanthomata in patient with primary biliary cirrhosis.

the latter for triglyceride synthesis. Withdrawal of alcohol results in a rapid decrease in triglyceride levels.

As illustrated in Table 10.1, an increased level of HDL cholesterol is a commoner consequence of regular heavy consumption of alcohol than is hypertriglyceridaemia; however, concomitant elevation of both lipids together with a raised γ-glutamyl transpeptidase is pathognomonic. The increase in HDL cholesterol reflects increases in both HDL_2 and HDL_3, the former being due to the increase in lipoprotein lipase activity which accompanies regular drinking.

10

Table 10.1 Characteristics of occasional versus heavy drinkers (median values).

	Occasional (n = 17)	Heavy (n = 19)	P^*
Age (years)	46	46	NS
Alcohol (units/week)	6	78	< 0.001
Gamma-glutamyl (iu/l) transferase	25	81	< 0.002
Cholesterol (mmol/l)	6.3	6.6	NS
Triglyceride (mmol/l)	1.39	1.47	NS
HDL-cholesterol (mmol/l)	1.1	1.5	< 0.005

*Mann-Whitney U-test. Data from Allaway *et al.*, *J R Soc Med* 1988, 81:149–151.

Rarely, excessively heavy drinking can give rise to Zieve's syndrome of jaundice, hyperlipaemia and haemolysis. In one series serum triglycerides ranged from 3 to 327 mmol/l, with a type V pattern in 40% of patients [20].

Dioxin and chlorinated hydrocarbons
Exposure to dioxin, the industrial toxin released in the Seveso disaster, gives rise to a syndrome characterized by chloracne, hirsutism, neurological dam-

age and hypercholesterolaemia [21]. It is possible that the latter is secondary to dioxin-mediated hypothyroidism but this remains to be shown. Chlorinated hydrocarbons such as the insecticide DDT can markedly elevate HDL cholesterol.

Iatrogenic

Numerous drugs have been shown to induce or aggravate hyperlipidaemia. Probably the most important group are drugs used to treat hypertension and angina, especially the thiazide diuretics and beta blockers. Evidence that treatment of hypertension did not have the expected beneficial effect on CHD has focused attention on the hyperlipidaemic properties of these commonly used drugs and led to suggestions that alternative drugs, which do not have this side-effect, should be used instead. These include angiotensin-converting enzyme (ACE) inhibitors, calcium antagonists and alpha$_1$ blockers [22]. Next in importance come immunosuppressive drugs, particularly corticosteroids and cyclosporin, which are used extensively in patients undergoing renal or cardiac transplantation, in whom persistent hyperlipidaemia may compromise the survival of the donor organ.

Antihypertensives
The effects of the various antihypertensive drugs in current use on serum lipids and lipoproteins are summarized in Table 10.2.

Administration of thiazide diuretics such as chlorthalidone and hydrochlorothiazide has long been recognized to increase total cholesterol and triglyceride. HDL cholesterol remains unaltered but VLDL and LDL cholesterol both increase. These changes probably reflect the adverse effects of these drugs on glucose tolerance and tend to be accompanied by hyperuricaemia. The effects, which are most marked in obese males and post-menopausal females, can be minimized by weight reduction and adherence to a modified fat diet. Spironolactone, indipamide, angiotensin converting enzyme inhibitors and calcium antagonists appear to have no adverse effects on serum lipids.

10

Long-term administration of beta blockers without intrinsic sympathomimetic activity (ISA) to patients with hypertension or CHD is associated with 15–30% increases in serum triglyceride and 6–8% decreases in HDL cholesterol. There appears to be little or no difference between non-selective drugs such as propranolol and cardioselective drugs such as atenolol in this respect [23]. However, beta blockers with ISA have a much less marked influence on serum lipids, and alpha blockers cause an increase in HDL cholesterol.

The mechanism of the hypertriglyceridaemic and HDL lowering effects of beta blockers is unclear but may involve a decrease in lipoprotein lipase due

Table 10.2. Effects of antihypertensive drugs on serum lipids and lipoproteins.

	TC	TG	HDLC	LDLC
Diuretics				
Thiazide	↑	↑	→	↑
Spironolactone	±	±		
Indapamide	±	±		
Beta blockers				
Without ISA	→	↑	↓	→
With ISA	→	→	→	→
α + β	→	→	→	→
Sympatholytics				
Prazosin	↓	→	±	↓
Clonidine	↓	→	→	↓
Methyldopa	→	→	→	→
ACE inhibitors	→	→	→	→
Calcium antagonists	→	→	→	→

ACE, angiotensin converting enzyme; TC, total cholesterol; TG, triglycerides; HDLC, high-density lipoprotein cholesterol; LDLC, low-density lipoprotein cholesterol; ISA, intrinsic sympathomimetic activity. Published by permission from Chobanian, *Am J Cardiol* 1987, 59:48F–52F.

to inhibition of adenyl cyclase in adipocytes. There is evidence that removal of triglycerides from plasma is impaired during beta blockade and this can lead to marked increases in serum triglyceride in individuals with a genetic predisposition to hypertriglyceridaemia, as illustrated in Fig. 10.6. This possibility, together with the apparent absence of any impact on CHD in hypertensives, should make clinicians think twice before prescribing a beta blocker as long-term treatment for hypertension or angina in a patient who is already hyperlipidaemic.

Immunosuppressants

Corticosteroids cause insulin resistance and impaired glucose tolerance, which leads to hypertriglyceridaemia and a reduction in HDL cholesterol. These abnormalities were commonly seen in renal transplant patients who were on high doses of steroids before cyclosporin was developed. Experimental studies suggest that a steroid-induced increase in VLDL synthesis is one of the mechanisms involved. Similar changes can occur spontaneously in patients with Cushing's syndrome.

Studies in renal transplant patients on cyclosporin show that this drug causes an increase in serum cholesterol, reflecting an increase in LDL cholesterol. It

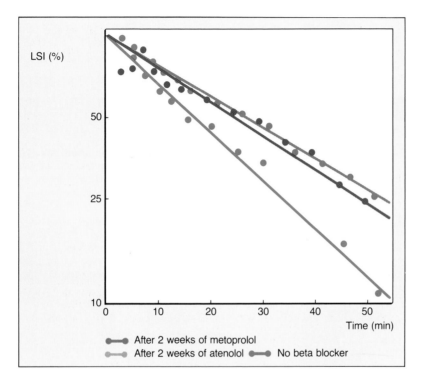

Fig. 10.6. Effect of beta blockers on light scattering index (LSI) after intravenous Intralipid in a patient with an apoE$_2$/E$_3$ phentoype, who had previously developed type V hyperlipoproteinaemia and acute pancreatitis while on metoprolol. Adapted by permission from Durrington and Cairns, *Br Med J* 1982, 284:1016.

10

has been suggested that the latter stems from a hepatotoxic effect of the drug, which results in impaired receptor-mediated LDL catabolism. Similar abnormalities occur in patients receiving steroids and cyclosporin after cardiac transplantation, especially those with a background of CHD.

Other drugs

An increase in HDL cholesterol has been well documented in epileptics receiving phenytoin [24]. A similar effect has been reported with barbiturates and with cimetidine, but not ranitidine. Cimetidine has also been reported to cause severe chylomicronaemia. Retinoids, which are used in dermatology, induce a marked increase in serum triglycerides, especially in patients with pre-existing type IV hyperlipoproteinaemia [25]. Undoubtedly there are many other iatrogenic influences not listed here which can cause hyperlipidaemia in certain individuals. Whenever this is suspected the drug in question should be temporarily discontinued and the effect of this on serum lipids should be assessed.

Miscellaneous causes

Over 50% of patients with anorexia nervosa are hypercholesterolaemic, because of marked increases in LDL [26]. Possible reasons are a high intake of dietary cholesterol in the form of eggs and cheese, or alternatively decreased LDL catabolism, as occurs after prolonged fasting in certain animals.

The presence of abnormal immunoglobulins in the circulation which bind to lipoproteins, enzymes or receptors can give rise to various types of secondary hyperlipidaemia including type I in systemic lupus erythematosus and type III in myelomatosis. An increase in LDL is a feature of acute intermittent porphyria whereas type V hyperlipoproteinaemia has been reported as a consequence of repetitive venesection for polycythaemia.

Annotated references

1.   KWITEROVICH PO, MARGOLIS S: Type IV hyperlipoproteinaemia. *Clin Endocrinol Metab* 1973, 2:41–71.
Dated but comprehensive review of the various causes, mechanisms and treatment of type IV hyperlipoproteinaemia.

2.   MABUCHI H, SAKAI Y, WATANABE A, HABA T, KOIZUMI J, TAKEDA R: Normalization of low-density lipoprotein levels and disappearance of xanthomas during pregnancy in a women with heterozygous familial hypercholesterolemia. *Metabolism* 1985, 34:309–316.
Unique case report of Japanese patient with FH who was studied during two pregnancies.

3.   WALLACE RB, HOOVER J, BARRETT-CONNOR E, RIFKIND B, HUNNINGHAKE DB, MACKENTHUN A, HEISS G: Altered plasma lipid and lipoprotein levels associated with oral contraceptive and oestrogen use. *Lancet* 1979, ii:111–115.
Comparison of effects on serum lipids of oral contraceptives in young women and oestrogen use in older women.

4.   MOLITCH ME, OILL P, ODELL WD: Massive hyperlipemia during estrogen therapy. *JAMA* 1974, 227:522–525.
Four examples of severe hypertriglyceridaemia in women on oral contraceptives or oestrogen replacement therapy.

10

5. FFRENCH-CONSTANT CK, SPENGEL FA, THOMPSON GR: Hyperlipidaemia and premature coronary disease following sex-change. *Postgrad Med J* 1985, 61:61–63.
Case report of hyperlipidaemia and coronary disease in female who underwent bilateral oophorectomy and took androgens.

6. SERIES JJ, BIGGART EM, O'REILLY D ST J, PACKARD CJ, SHEPHERD J: Thyroid dysfunction and hypercholesterolaemia in the general population of Glasgow, Scotland. *Clin Chim Acta* 1988, 172:217–222.
Useful survey of the prevalence of hypothyroidism among hypercholesterolaemic individuals.

7. HOWARD BV: Lipoprotein metabolism in diabetes mellitus. *J Lipid Res* 1987, 28:613–628.
Comprehensive review of lipid and lipoprotein metabolism in juvenile and maturity onset diabetes.

8. STEINER G: Diabetes and atherosclerosis: an overview. *Diabetes* 1981, 30 (suppl 2):1–7.
Brief, helpful review of the pathogenesis of atherosclerosis in diabetics.

9. SIMPSON HCR, SIMPSON RW, LOUSLEY S, CARTER RD, GEEKIE M, HOCKADAY TDR, MANN JI: A high carbohydrate leguminous fibre diet improves all aspects of diabetic control. *Lancet* 1981, i:1–5.
Comparison of high-carbohydrate, high-fibre and low-carbohydrate diets in patients with insulin-dependent and non-insulin-dependent diabetes.

10. REAVEN GM: Abnormal lipoprotein metabolism in non-insulin-dependent diabetes mellitus. *Am J Med* 1987, 83 (suppl 3A):31–40.
Detailed appraisal of the causation and management of hyperlipidaemia in maturity onset diabetes, including the role of insulin resistance.

11. GARG A, GRUNDY SM: Treatment of dyslipidemia in non-insulin-dependent diabetes mellitus with lovastatin. *Am J Cardiol* 1988, 62:44J–49J.
Assessment of the value of lovastatin in the treatment of hyperlipidaemia in 16 patients with NIDDM.

12. BLUESTONE R, LEWIS B, MERVART I: Hyperlipoproteinaemia in gout. *Ann Rheum Dis* 1971, 30:134–137.
Clinical description of the frequent occurrence of hypertriglyceridaemia in primary gout.

13. ANGEL A, RONCARI DAK: Medical complications of obesity. *Can Med Assoc J* 1978, 119:1408–1411.
Appraisal of the cardiovascular consequences of obesity by two experts in the field.

14. KESANIEMI YA, GRUNDY SM: Increased low density lipoprotein production associated with obesity. *Arteriosclerosis* 1983, 3:170–177.
Comparative studies of LDL-apoB turnover and cholesterol balance in normal and obese men.

10

15.   BENNETT WM, BARDANA EJ, WUEPPER K, HOUGHTON D, BORDER WA, GOTZE O, SCHREIBER R: **Partial lipodystrophy, C3 nephritic factor and clinically inapparent mesangiocapillary glomerulonephritis.** *Am J Med* 1977, 62:757–760.
Description of female with partial lipodystrophy associated with type IV hyperlipoproteinaemia and subclinical renal involvement.

16.   JÜNGST D, CASELMANN WH, KUTSCHERA P, WEISWEILER P: **Relation of hyperlipidemia in serum and loss of high density lipoproteins in urine in the nephrotic syndrome.** *Clin Chim Acta* 1987, 168:159–167.
Studies of lipoprotein abnormalities in 19 patients with the nephrotic syndrome, including the relative importance of urinary excretion of albumin and HDL.

17.   NESTEL PJ, FIDGE NH, TAN MH: **Increased lipoprotein remnant formation in chronic renal failure.** *N Engl J Med* 1982, 307:329–333.
Detailed analysis of the lipoprotein abnormalities seen in haemodialysed patients which showed increased formation and accumulation of remnant particles in plasma.

18.   NICHOLLS AJ, CUMMING AM, CATTO GRD, EDWARD N, ENGESET J: **Lipid relationships in dialysis and renal transplant patients.** *Q J Med* 1981, 50:149–160.
Comparison of lipoprotein changes observed in 28 patients undergoing haemodialysis and in 20 patients following renal transplant.

19.   SEIDEL D, ALAUPOVIC P, FURMAN RH, MCCONATHY WJ: **A lipoprotein characterizing obstructive jaundice.** *J Clin Invest* 1970, 49:2396.
First description of Lp-X.

20.   BENRAAD HB, PENN JH, PIETERS GFFM, TAN HS: **Zieve's syndrome.** *J R Coll Phys* 1977, 12:42–52.
Description of the clinical and biochemical features of 11 patients with Zieve's syndrome.

21.   OLIVER RM: **Toxic effects of 2,3,7,8 tetrachlorodibenzo 1,4 dioxin in laboratory workers.** *Br J Ind Med* 1975, 32:49–53.
Case report of three scientists who were accidentally contaminated with dioxin and developed symptoms and signs of toxicity 2–3 years later.

22.   DZAU VJ: **Recommendations of the Adult Treatment Panel of the National Cholesterol Education Program. Implications for the management of hypertension.** *Hypertension* 1988, 12:471–473.
Thoughtful appraisal of new attitudes to the choice of antihypertensive drugs in the light of recent recommendations about desirable levels of blood cholesterol.

23.   MILLER NE: **Effects of adrenoceptor-blocking drugs on plasma lipoprotein concentrations.** *Am J Cardiol* 1987, 60:17E–23E.
Useful and objective analysis of the effects on serum lipids of the various classes of antihypertensive drugs.

24.   NIKKILA E, KASTE M, ENHOLM C, VIIKARI J: **Increase of serum high density lipoprotein in phenytoin users.** *Br Med J* 1978, 2:99.
Description of raised levels of HDL cholesterol and apoA-I attributed to use of the anticonvulsant drug, phenytoin.

10

25.   KATZ RA, JORGENSEN H, NIGRA TH: **Elevation of serum triglyceride levels from oral isotretinoin in disorders of keratinization.** *Arch Dermatol* 1980, 116:1369–1372.
Early description of the hypertriglyceridaemic effects of retinoids.

26.   MORDASINI R, KLOSE G, GRETEN H: **Secondary type II hyperlipoproteinaemia in patients with anorexia nervosa.** *Metabolism* 1978, 27:71–79.
Anorexia nervosa is frequently accompanied by increases in LDL cholesterol.

10

11 MANAGEMENT OF HYPERLIPIDAEMIA

Pros and cons of lipid-lowering

Investigation of the hyperlipidaemic patient
History
Clinical examination
Laboratory tests

Dietary therapy
Modified fat diets
Vegetable protein and fibre
AHA and NCEP recommendations
Pregnancy, lactation and infancy

Physical exercise

Control of other risk factors

Role of the lipid clinic

Annotated references

Pros and cons of lipid-lowering

Before discussing the practical management of hyperlipidaemia it makes sense first to define the objectives to be achieved. These will vary according to the type of hyperlipidaemia and its severity. For example, the object of treating those types of hyperlipidaemia associated with chylomicronaemia is to reduce triglyceride levels, sufficiently to prevent the occurrence of acute pancreatitis. On the other hand the main reason for treating types of hyperlipidaemia characterized by increases in VLDL, IDL and LDL is to decrease the level of these atherogenic lipoproteins and at the same time increase the level of anti-atherogenic HDL, so as to minimize the risk of vascular disease. In this context the degree of cholesterol-lowering to be achieved will depend upon whether one is embarking on primary prevention in an asymptomatic individual or secondary intervention in a patient with established disease.

In patients with CHD the potential benefits of lipid-lowering therapy outweigh the risks of side effects. However, in asymptomatic subjects at increased risk of CHD the possible risks of lipid-lowering therapy must be carefully considered before embarking on lifelong treatment, especially if this necessitates the use of drugs.

One of the best documented side effects of treatment is the lithogenic effect of clofibrate, which resulted in a doubling of the incidence of gallstones during the WHO trial [1] and the Coronary Drug project [2]. This undoubtedly contributed to the increase in non-cardiovascular mortality observed in the WHO trial, if only because it reflected the high fatality rate associated with cholecystectomy in some parts of Europe. Cholesterol-lowering diets high in polyunsaturated fat probably also predispose to gallstones [3]. There is also concern about the apparent relationship between low serum cholesterol levels and cancer. Initially it was thought that this simply reflected the fact that hypocholesterolaemia is an early sign of an occult neoplasm [4], but recent studies cast doubt on this as the sole explanation [5,6]. Although lacking statistical significance, there was a tendency in both the MRFIT and Coronary Primary Prevention Trials for certain gastrointestinal tract neoplasms to be more common among treated subjects. More data are needed to resolve this important question.

With these provisos in mind and in view of the long-term nature of lipid-lowering therapy it should be evident that an all-out commitment to this endeavour, by whatever means prove necessary, should be reserved for patients with established atherosclerotic complications or for those known to have a high risk of developing them, as defined in Chapter 14. Evidence that effective intervention beneficially influences CHD in these two categories is reviewed in the same chapter.

Investigation of the hyperlipidaemic patient

11

This section deals with the investigation of individuals shown to be hyperlipidaemic on at least one fasting blood sample, and who have been subsequently referred to a lipid clinic. Often this will require only two visits and subsequent management at follow-up can be undertaken by the referring practitioner.

History
History taking is as important here as in every other branch of medicine. Hyperlipidaemia *per se* seldom causes symptoms (excepting Achilles tendonitis in FH) but attempts should be made to elicit any symptoms of vascular insufficiency, such as angina, claudication or transient ischaemic attacks, or a history of severe abdominal pain suggestive of an episode of acute pancreatitis. The past history should include details of any previous measurement of serum lipids, so as to help establish the duration of hyperlipidaemia, and of

any complications such as myocardial infarction, or surgical procedures such as coronary artery bypass grafting, angioplasty or cholecystectomy. A history of diabetes, thyroid dysfunction, gout and renal disease is also relevant.

Family history is of great importance, especially the age of onset or death from coronary heart disease of relatives. A family history of hyperlipidaemia and other risk factors should also be sought, including hypertension, diabetes and gout. Construction of a family tree will help in screening all those at risk.

The patient's social history should include details of occupation and marital status, age and sex of children, and whether they have been tested for hyperlipidaemia, and also dietary habits including alcohol and sucrose consumption, current and past smoking habits, amount of exercise taken and current drug history.

Clinical examination
It is important to undertake a full physical examination during the patient's first visit, paying particular attention to whether there are any external signs of hyperlipidaemia, such as corneal arcus, xanthelasma or xanthomata. Places to examine are the palms of the hands for palmar striae, elbows, knees and buttocks for eruptive xanthomata, and the dorsum of the hands and feet, pretibial tuberosities and Achilles tendons for tendon xanthomata. Other signs which should be sought are aortic murmurs, reduced or absent pulses in the limbs, carotid bruits and the presence of any retinopathy.

Examination of the abdomen should include assessment of liver size and presence of splenomegaly. Endocrine status should also be briefly considered, in particular whether there is any evidence of hypothyroidism or Cushing's syndrome. The blood pressure should always be measured and the urine tested for the presence of protein, glucose and blood.

11

Laboratory tests
The most important of these is to confirm the presence of hyperlipidaemia in serum or plasma obtained after an overnight fast of over 10 hours duration. Measurements to be undertaken should include total cholesterol, triglyceride and HDL cholesterol, with calculation of LDL cholesterol and HDL ratio as described in earlier chapters. If possible measurements of apoB, apoA-I and Lp(a) should also be performed. Examination of hyperlipaemic plasma or serum left standing overnight at 4°C, lipoprotein electrophoresis and apoE phenotyping are useful in helping to differentiate between types I, III and V hyperlipoproteinaemia. More esoteric tests include agar gel electrophoresis to detect Lp-X, measurement of post-heparin lipolytic and LCAT activities, and analysis of the fatty acid composition of cholesterol esters in plasma. The latter investigations and also ultracentrifugal isolation of lipoproteins re-

quire access to facilities which ordinarily exist only in a research laboratory or teaching hospital.

In addition to characterizing the severity and nature of the patient's hyperlipidaemia a search should be made for underlying causes of secondary hyperlipidaemia. Routinely this involves undertaking a full biochemical profile including tests of renal and hepatic function, fasting glucose and thyroid function tests (T4 and TSH). Additional investigations which may be required are γ-glutamyl transpeptidase, as an index of alcohol intake, a protein electrophoretic strip to determine the presence of paraproteinaemia, and measurement of creatine phosphokinase (CPK) if a myositic syndrome is suspected in a patient undergoing treatment with lipid-lowering drugs.

Other investigations which should be done routinely at the first visit are measurement of height and weight, the latter being repeated at every subsequent attendance, and a resting electrocardiogram.

Dietary therapy

It is a truism that dietary modification is the corner stone of any lipid-lowering regimen. Often diet alone will be successful in controlling hyperlipidaemia, especially where this is due mainly to a faulty diet or obesity. However, diet can be beneficial even in genetically determined forms of hyperlipidaemia and if drugs are required they should be given in addition to rather than instead of a lipid-lowering diet.

Obesity is a prime cause of hyperlipidaemia, especially hypertriglyceridaemia, and one of the most important accessories required by the lipidologist is a set of tables specifying the desirable range of weight in relation to height for both men and women, e.g. 1983 Metropolitan Height and Mass Tables [7]. It is essential to weigh all patients at their first attendance and to indicate the extent to which their weight differs from the ideal value, which is based on the lowest mortality of insured persons aged 25–59 in the USA.

Ideally dietary advice should be provided by a qualified dietician or nutritionist, who will start by assessing the patient's intake of total energy, protein, carbohydrate and fat, including its P : S ratio and cholesterol content. Alcohol consumption should also be estimated. Having carried out this assessment the dietician will then be able to advise the patient and the patient's spouse on the quantitative and qualitative changes in diet needed to achieve ideal body weight and optimal serum lipids.

11

Modified fat diets

Generally speaking modified fat diets differ from 'normal' diets in containing less total fat, saturated fat and cholesterol, and more polyunsaturated fat. Protein intake is kept fairly constant so that relatively more of the total energy intake is derived from carbohydrate, specifically complex carbohydrate rather than refined sugars. The amount of energy provided should be just sufficient to enable the patient to achieve and maintain desirable body weight. The overall impact of such changes on lipoprotein metabolism and the importance of body weight in regulating cholesterol synthesis have been reviewed in detail recently by McNamara [8].

The 1973 National Food Survey showed that on average Britons consumed 2400 calories daily, of which 46% was carbohydrate, 12% was protein and 42% was fat, with a P : S ratio of 0.23 and a cholesterol content of 500 mg. Half the fat came from dairy produce. In contrast, a typical modified fat diet provides up to 2000 calories per day, of which 52% is carbohydrate, 16% protein and 32% fat, with a P : S ratio of 1.5, and less than 300 mg cholesterol. Such a diet is effective in the treatment of both hypercholesterolaemia and hypertriglyceridaemia [9].

Most subjects show obvious decreases in serum lipids and a rise in the HDL ratio after 6–12 weeks on a modified fat diet, as exemplified in Table 11.1. Failure to respond usually indicates either non-compliance, which can be monitored by measuring the linoleate content of plasma lipids or adipose tissue, or genuine non-responsiveness. Occurrence of the latter phenomenon despite achievement of desirable body weight suggests a genetic basis for the hyperlipidaemia, such as FH or FCH.

Table 11.1. Effects of a 2000-calorie modified fat diet for 6 weeks in 11 male control subjects.

Variable	Before	After	P
Body weight (kg)	74.8 ± 8.3	71.7 ± 7.8	< 0.001
Serum cholesterol (mmol/l)	6.0 ± 0.8	5.0 ± 0.6	< 0.001
Serum triglyceride (mmol/l)	1.4 ± 0.6	1.0 ± 0.5	< 0.001
HDL cholesterol (mmol/l)	1.1 ± 0.3	1.1 ± 0.2	NS
HDL ratio	0.24 ± 0.09	0.30 ± 0.09	< 0.01
Plasma triglyceride, % 18:2 (n = 8)	14.8 ± 3.9	27.0 ± 7.1	< 0.01

Published by permission from Thompson, in *Lipoproteins, Atherosclerosis and Coronary Heart Disease* edited by Miller and Lewis. Amsterdam: Elsevier-North Holland, 1981, pp 129–143.

11

Despite their higher carbohydrate content modified fat diets are more effective than low carbohydrate diets in reducing VLDL levels and controlling hypertriglyceridaemia [10]. They are also effective in reducing LDL cholesterol but this is often accompanied by a decrease in HDL cholesterol if the total fat content is very low or if the P : S ratio is above 2 [11]. Modified fat diets containing 30–35% total fat with a P : S ratio of 1.0 do not have this potentially undesirable effect [12]. Also, substitution of monounsaturated oleate for saturated fat is as effective as polyunsaturated linoleate in reducing LDL cholesterol but does not reduce HDL cholesterol [13].

The cholesterol-lowering effect of reducing dietary cholesterol is debatable, unless the intake is very high [8], but it makes sense to patients whereas a negative attitude is confusing, especially to those with FH. Alcohol has a beneficial effect on HDL cholesterol when taken regularly in moderation and need not be proscribed. However, excessive amounts induce hypertriglyceridaemia in some patients, as can be assessed by asking them to abstain from all alcohol for at least 1 week prior to the taking of their next blood sample.

Patients with types I and V hyperlipoproteinaemia are exceptionally sensitive to long-chain dietary fat which should be restricted to 30–50 g/day, so as to avoid acute pancreatitis, but medium-chain triglyceride is allowed. Alcohol consumption must also be strictly limited since it stimulates VLDL synthesis, thereby imposing an extra load on triglyceride-clearing mechanisms and aggravating hyperchylomicronaemia. Patients with type IV hyperlipoproteinaemia responding incompletely to a modified fat diet may benefit from total avoidance of sucrose. Excessive consumption of coffee, especially if boiled, should be avoided in hypercholesterolaemic patients, as discussed in Chapter 1.

Vegetable protein and fibre

Several studies have shown that substituting vegetable protein for animal protein in the diet results in a fall in serum cholesterol, despite the fat and cholesterol content of the diet being kept constant. Substitution of soybean protein for animal protein led to a 25% decrease in serum cholesterol in type II patients, including some with FH [14]. The mechanism of this effect is uncertain but the observation itself might explain why some populations in the Far East, where animal protein intake is less than in the West, have lower serum cholesterol levels than would be expected from the fat and cholesterol content of their diet. Vegetarians have lower serum lipids than non-vegetarians but it is probable that this is only partly attributable to the source of protein, in view of the high P : S ratio and low cholesterol content of vegetarian diets.

Certain types of soluble fibre cause an increase in faecal bile acid excretion and thereby exert a cholesterol-lowering effect. Thus the ingestion of 13 g of guar daily as crispbread by type II and IV patients resulted in 13% decreases in serum cholesterol and triglyceride [15] whereas 100 g of oat-bran per day in the form of cereal and muffins induced a 14% decrease in LDL cholesterol [16]. Insoluble fibre in the form of cellulose had no such effect.

The value of beans, peas and lentils as a suitable source of food in the treatment of hyperlipidaemia is becoming increasingly recognized, especially those varieties which are rich in vegetable protein and soluble fibre. The main

11

limitation of this type of diet is its tendency to cause gastrointestinal side effects, the most noticeable of which is excessive flatulence.

AHA and NCEP recommendations

The 1984 American Heart Association (AHA) guidelines for the treatment of hyperlipidaemia in adults have recently been reviewed by Grundy [17] who played a key role in their formulation. These advocate that patients with mild hypercholesterolaemia be advised to follow the AHA phase I diet, which is also recommended for the American population at large. The main features of this modified fat diet are shown in Table 11.2. If the response is poor or if the patient has other risk factors then the AHA phase II should be tried (Table 11.3). Patients with severe or unresponsive hypercholesterolaemia may need to go to the AHA phase III diet (Table 11.4). Mild, moderate and severe hypercholesterolaemia were defined by Grundy as serum cholesterol levels in the ranges 5.2–6.5, 6.5–7.8 and >7.8 mmol/l, respectively. Similar recommendations have been made by the European Atherosclerosis Society [18].

Even more recent guidelines for dietary therapy of hypercholesterolaemia were promulgated as part of the National Cholesterol Education Program (NCEP) in the USA [19]. These recommendations have been summarized by Hatcher *et al.* [20], as shown in Table 11.5. In essence the NCEP step-one and step-two diets correspond to the AHA phase I and phase II diets. These diets are considered suitable for treating all types of hyperlipidaemia with the exception of type I, where more drastic restriction of fat intake may be necessary.

Reductions of serum cholesterol of between 0.5 and 1.5 mmol/l should be achievable with these diets. This effect is usually evident within 3 months but if not then diet should be maintained for at least 6 months all told before considering the addition of a lipid-lowering drug. An exception should be made for patients known to have FH or severe hypercholesterolaemia (>7.8 mmol/l), where drug therapy is usually necessary and can be started sooner.

11

Pregnancy, lactation and infancy

All serum lipids tend to increase in pregnancy but return to baseline within 2 months of parturition. There is no reason why a modified fat diet should not be maintained by hyperlipidaemic patients during pregnancy and lactation as long as it has a P:S ratio of at least 1.0. Hormonal changes during pregnancy can aggravate hypertriglyceridaemia and it may be necessary to restrict fat intake to below 10% in those at risk of pancreatitis. AHA guidelines for children with FH between the ages of 1 and 10 years include reducing fat intake to 25–30% of total calories, with a P:S ratio of 1, and a cholesterol content of <200 mg per day. After cessation of breast-feeding infants should preferably be fed on a milk formula which contains polyunsaturated fat rather than butterfat. Some recommend that whole cow's milk should be used sub-

Table 11.2. American Heart Association Recommended Diet (phase I).

Composition
Limit fat intake to 30% of total calories with a sat:mono:poly ratio of 1:1:1,
dietary cholesterol less than 300 mg/day

General description
Limit meat to no more than 200 g (7 oz)/day
— Use fish and poultry more frequently than other meats.
— Include only chicken and turkey with skin removed.
— Any fatty fish (e.g. salmon) is acceptable for phase I.
— Use lean cuts of veal, beef, pork or lamb.

Restrict whole eggs to two per week, including those used in cooking (egg
white may be used as desired).

Restrict milk products to 1% fat milk, ice sorbets, low-fat yogurt, low-fat
cheese and low-fat cottage cheese.

Avoid hard fats such as butter, regular cheeses, lard, coconut oil, palm oil,
chocolates; use only vegetable oils, olive oil or soft-tub margarines.

Bread, cereals, pasta, potatoes and rice are allowed, except when made with
egg yolks.

Avoid whole-milk products, marbled meats, fish eggs, organ meats, bakery
goods made with hard fats and egg yolks, and rich desserts.

Published by permission [17].

sequently rather than skimmed milk because of the former's importance as
a major source of calories and fat-soluble vitamins [21].

11   Physical exercise

Numerous studies have shown that moderate amounts of aerobic exercise
(walking, jogging, swimming, cycling or cross-country skiing) on a regular basis have beneficial effects on serum lipids. These include reductions in serum
triglyceride and LDL cholesterol and increases in lipoprotein lipase activity
and HDL cholesterol, especially HDL_2. Significant effects were observed within
2 months in middle-aged men exercising for 30 min thrice weekly [22]. In
joggers the decrease in LDL cholesterol has been shown to be proportional to
the distance run, as shown in Fig. 11.1, but it is necessary to run over 10 miles
per week before significant changes in HDL cholesterol are observed. However, lesser amounts of exercise are effective in reducing triglyceride levels in
type IV patients. Obviously the amount of exercise which can be taken will
depend upon whether the individuals involved have CHD but within reason

Table 11.3. American Heart Association Recommended Diet (phase II).

Composition
Limit fat intake to 25% of total calories with a sat:mono:poly ratio of 1:1:1, dietary cholesterol less than 200 mg/day

General description
Limit meat to no more than 170 g (6 oz)/day.
— Restrict red meat in favour of fish and poultry.
— Use chicken and turkey with skin removed and use lean cuts of meat only.

Eat no egg yolks, although egg whites and substitutes may be used.

Restrict milk products to $^1/_2$ % fat milk, ice sorbets, low fat cheese and low-fat cottage cheese.

Avoid hard fats such as butter, regular cheeses, lard, coconut oil, palm oil, chocolates; use only vegetable oils, olive oil or soft-tub margarines.

All vegetables and fruits are allowed except for coconut; limit olives and avocadoes.

Bread, cereals, pasta, potatoes and rice are allowed, except when made with egg yolks; limit starchy foods to prevent weight gain.

Avoid whole-milk products, marbled meats, fish eggs, organ meats, bakery goods made with hard fats and egg yolks, and rich desserts.

Published by permission [17].

all hyperlipidaemic patients should be encouraged to take as much as feasible. The VLDL-reducing and HDL-raising effects of exercise are accentuated by dietary modification and by weight loss in those who are overweight.

Control of other risk factors   11

Treatment of hyperlipidaemia should always be accompanied by detection and control of any other risk factors which may be present. This is important on two counts, firstly because certain risk factors such as diabetes can aggravate hyperlipidaemia, and secondly because the risk of CHD is accentuated when several risk factors co-exist.

Obesity, hypertension and smoking all aggravate the cardiovascular consequences of hyperlipidaemia, albeit by different mechanisms. Their control or elimination needs to be achieved if lipid-lowering therapy is to be fully effective. The choice of antihypertensive drugs should take into consideration that diuretics and beta blockers can have adverse effects on serum lipids whereas

Table 11.4. American Heart Association Recommended Diet (phase III).

Composition
Limit fat intake to 20% of total calories with a sat:mono:poly ratio of 1:1:1, dietary cholesterol less than 150 mg/day

General description
Limit meat to 85 g (3 oz)/day.
— Restrict red meat in favour of fish and poultry.
— Use chicken and turkey with skin removed and use lean cuts.
of meat only.

Use no egg yolks, although egg whites and substitutes may be used.

Restrict milk products to skimmed milk, skimmed-milk yogurt, and cheese with less than 1% fat.

Avoid hard fats; use only small quantities of vegetable oils, olive oil or soft-tub margarines.

All vegetables and fruits are allowed except for coconut, olives and avocadoes.

Cereals, pasta, potatoes, rice and fat-free bread are allowed, except when made with egg yolks.

Avoid whole-milk products, marbled meats, fish eggs, organ meats, bakery goods made with hard fats and egg yolks, and rich desserts.

Published by permission [17].

11

Table 11.5. Dietary therapy of hypercholesterolaemia.

Nutrient	Step-one diet	Step-two diet
Total fat*	Less than 30%	Less than 30%
Fatty acids*		
Saturated	Less than 10%	Less than 7%
Polyunsaturated	Up to 10%	Up to 10%
Monounsaturated	10–15%	10–15%
Carbohydrates*	50–60%	50–60%
Protein*	10–20%	10–20%
Cholesterol	Less than 300 mg/day	Less than 200 mg/day
Total calories	To achieve and maintain desirable weight	To achieve and maintain desirable weight

*Per cent of total calories. Published by permission [20].

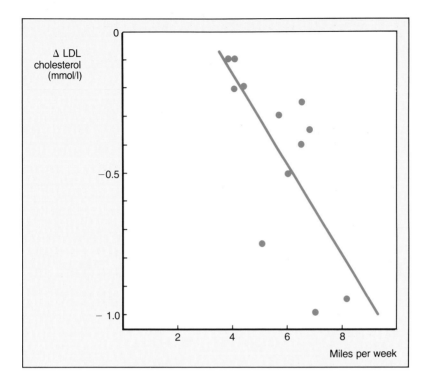

Fig. 11.1. Correlation between change in LDL cholesterol and distance run in 12 subjects during 6 weeks of exercise ($r = 0.74$, $P < 0.01$). Adapted by permission from Kaufman *et al.*, *Artery* 1980, 7:99–108.

11

calcium antagonists and ACE inhibitors appear to be free from this disadvantage.

Control of hyperglycaemia by diet, oral hypoglycaemic agents or insulin should be as good as possible. However, despite this hyperlipidaemia can often be a persistent problem in diabetics and may necessitate a lipid-lowering drug.

Oral contraceptives tend to increase serum triglycerides and decrease HDL cholesterol whereas the thrombogenic properties of oestrogens have been held responsible for cerebrovascular accidents in young women with FH. Oral contraceptives should be avoided or if this is not feasible safer preparations should be used such as progestogen-only pills containing desogestrel, but not levonorgestrel, or a combined preparation containing desogestrel and a low dose of ethinyl oestradiol. Post-menopausal hormone replacement therapy with oestrogens helps reduce LDL cholesterol and raise HDL in type II patients and reduce β-VLDL in type III patients but may aggravate hypertriglyceridaemia in those with type IV or V hyperlipoproteinaemia. Oestrogen cutaneous patches seem free from this tendency and should be used instead.

Role of the lipid clinic

The management of hyperlipidaemia is often best initiated in a hospital-based lipid clinic, especially if it has failed to respond to simple dietary measures. The chief advantages of a lipid clinic are availability of specialist advice and laboratory facilities, ease of cardiological referral, and the availability of dieticians, pharmacists and a research nurse, who can undertake the screening of other family members. Patients with FH and severe forms of hyperlipidaemia are best followed up permanently in a lipid clinic but most other patients can be returned to the care of their own general practitioner once the diagnosis has been made and treatment successfully instituted. The aims of treatment will vary according to the type of hyperlipidaemia being treated and the presence or otherwise of atherosclerotic vascular disease. Intervals between follow-up visits range from bimonthly initially to 4–6 monthly once the hyperlipidaemia is under control.

Ideally a lipid clinic should be staffed by physicians with a special interest and training in lipidology, but such individuals are in short supply. A general medical background is highly desirable and it is also useful if there are other members of the team with expertise in cardiology, clinical biochemistry and genetics. At present lipid clinics are often run by endocrinologists with a special interest in diabetes or by chemical pathologists. In the future, the advent of new and potent lipid-lowering therapies which can influence the course of atherosclerosis should help stimulate cardiologists to take a greater interest in this subject than hitherto. The incorporation of a period of theoretical and practical tuition in lipidology into the training requirements of cardiologists would be an important step in that direction.

11

Annotated references

1.   COMMITTEE OF PRINCIPAL INVESTIGATORS: WHO cooperative trial on primary prevention of ischaemic heart disease using clofibrate to lower serum cholesterol:mortality follow-up. *Lancet* 1980, ii:379–385.
Four-year follow-up data from WHO clofibrate trial showing excess of non-cardiovascular deaths in treated group due to various causes including gall-bladder disease.

2.   THE CORONARY DRUG PROJECT RESEARCH GROUP: **Clofibrate and niacin in coronary heart disease.** *JAMA* 1975, 231:360–381.
Detailed report of effects of clofibrate and nicotinic acid during the Coronary Drug Project including a twofold increase in gallstones in those treated with the former drug.

3.   STURDEVANT RAL, PEARCE ML, DAYTON S: **Increased prevalence of cholelithiasis in men ingesting a serum-cholesterol-lowering diet.** *N Engl J Med* 1973, 288:24–27.
Post-mortem data from the Los Angeles Veterans Study showing an excess of gallstones in those who had been on the high P : S ratio diet.

4.   INTERNATIONAL COLLABORATIVE GROUP: **Circulating cholesterol level and risk of death from cancer in men aged 40 to 69 years.** *JAMA* 1982, 248:2853–2859.
Data which suggest that inverse correlation between serum cholesterol and cancer mortality in over 60 000 men in eight countries is due to metabolic effects of undetected tumours.

5.   SALMOND CE, BEAGLEHOLE R, PRIOR IAM: **Are low cholesterol values associated with excess mortality?** *Br Med J* 1985, 290:422–424.
Inverse correlation between serum cholesterol and deaths from cancer in Maoris persisted even after excluding deaths during first 5 years of follow-up, which suggests that preclinical tumours depressing the serum cholesterol is not the whole explanation.

6.   SCHATZKIN A, HOOVER RN, TAYLOR PR, ZIEGLER RG, CARTER CL, LARSON DB, LICITRA LM: **Serum cholesterol and cancer in the NHANES. 1. Epidemiologic follow-up study.** *Lancet* 1987, ii:298–301.
Ten-year follow-up of over 5000 men showed risk of cancer greatest in those with serum cholesterol in lowest quintile, measured over 6 years previously.

7.   LENTNER C (ED.): *Geigy Scientific Tables Vol 3 8th edn.* Basle: Ciba-Geigy, 1984.
Tables of desirable weight in relation to height that all those working in a lipid clinic should possess.

8.   MCNAMARA DJ: **Effects of fat-modified diets on cholesterol and lipoprotein metabolism.** *Annu Rev Nutr* 1987, 7:273–290.
Comprehensive and critical review of a complex and important topic.

9.   TABAQCHALI S, CHAIT A, HARRISON R, LEWIS B: **Experience with simplified scheme of treatment of hyperlipidaemia.** *Br Med J* 1974, 3:377–380.
Early report of beneficial effects of a modified fat diet in patients with either hypercholes-terolaemia or hypertriglyceridaemia.

10.   SOMMARIVA D, SCOTTI L, FASOLI A: **Low-fat diet versus low-carbohydrate diet in the treatment of type IV hyperlipoproteinaemia.** *Atherosclerosis* 1978, 29:43–51.
Study which shows that low-fat diet was more effective in reducing serum lipids than a low carbohydrate diet in patients with hypertriglyceridaemia.

11.   SCHAEFER EJ, LEVY RI, ERNST ND, VAN SANT FD, BREWER HB: **The effects of low cholesterol, high polyunsaturated fat, and low fat diets on plasma lipid and lipo-protein cholesterol levels in normal and hypercholesterolemic subjects.** *Am J Clin Nutr* 1981, 34:1758–1763.
Dietary study showing that high P : S ratio or very low fat diets reduce both HDL and LDL cholesterol to a similar extent, so that the ratio does not change.

11

12. JONES DB, LOUSLEY S, SLAUGHTER P, CARTER RD, MANN JI: **Prudent diet: effect on moderately severe hyperlipidaemia.** *Br Med J* 1982, **284**:1233.
Small-scale study of lipid-lowering effects of modified fat diet with P:S ratio of one in patients with type IIb and type IV hyperlipoproteinaemia showing increases in the HDL:LDL ratio.

13. MATTSON FH, GRUNDY SM: **Comparison of effects of dietary saturated, monounsaturated and polyunsaturated fatty acids on plasma lipids and lipoproteins in man.** *J Lipid Res* 1985, **26**:194–202.
Important liquid formula dietary study which demonstrates that monounsaturated and polyunsaturated fats lower LDL cholesterol to the same extent but that monounsaturated fats reduced HDL cholesterol less than polyunsaturated fats.

14. DESCOVICH GC, CEREDI C, GADDI A, BENASSI MS, MANNINO G, COLOMBO L, CATTIN L, FONTANA G, SENIN U, MANNARINO E, CARUZZO C, BERTELLI E, FRAGIACOMO C, NOSEDA G, SIRTORI M, SIRTORI CR: **Multicentre study of soybean protein diet for outpatient hypercholesterolaemic patients.** *Lancet* 1980, **ii**:709–712.
Incorporation of soybean protein into the Italian diet appears to be a feasible and useful means of increasing the LDL-lowering effects of a high P:S ratio diet.

15. JENKINS DJA, REYNOLDS D, SLAVIN B, LEEDS AR, JENKINS AL, JEPSON EM: **Dietary fiber and blood lipids: treatment of hypercholesterolemia with guar crispbread.** *Am J Clin Nutr* 1980, **33**:575–581.
Observations on the lipid-lowering and laxative effects of guar.

16. KIRBY RW, ANDERSON JW, SIELING B, REES ED, LIN CHEN W-J, MILLER RE, KAY RM: **Oat-bran intake selectively lowers serum low density lipoprotein cholesterol concentrations of hypercholesterolemic men.** *Am J Clin Nutr* 1981, **34**:824–829.
Demonstration of the lipid-lowering effects of oat-bran which vindicates the adage that porridge is good for you.

17. GRUNDY SM: **Dietary treatment of hyperlipidemia.** In *Hypercholesterolemia and Atherosclerosis. Pathogenesis and Prevention* edited by Steinberg D, Olefsky JM. New York: Churchill Livingstone 1987, pp 169–193.
Excellent review of the rationale and practical aspects of the dietary treatment of different types of hyperlipidaemia.

18. STUDY GROUP, EUROPEAN ATHEROSCLEROSIS SOCIETY: **Strategies for the prevention of coronary heart disease: a policy statement of the European Atherosclerosis Society.** *Eur Heart J* 1987, **8**:77–88.
A detailed statement on the detection and management of CHD compiled and promulgated under the aegis of the EAS.

19. THE EXPERT PANEL: **Report of the National Cholesterol Education Program Expert Panel on detection, evaluation and treatment of high blood cholesterol in adults.** *Arch Intern Med* 1988, **148**:36–69.
Very detailed description of the official position on the definition and management of hyperlipidaemia currently in the USA.

20. HATCHER LF, FLAVELL DP, ILLINGWORTH DR: **Dietary therapy of hypercholesterolemia.** *Practical Cardiology,* Special Issue, May 1988, pp 31–37.

11

A readable digest of the NCEP guidelines which also includes a lot of useful dietetic advice.

21.   BENTLEY D, LAWSON M: **Clinical nutrition in paediatric disorders.** London: Baillière Tindall, 1988.
Recent book on clinical nutrition with useful information for paediatricians involved in treating hyperlipidaemia.

22.   HUTTUNEN JK, LANSIMIES E, VOUTILAINEN E, ENHOLM C, HIETANEN E, PENTILLA I, SIITONEN O, RAURAMAA R: **Effect of moderate physical exercise on serum lipoproteins. A controlled clinical trial with special reference to serum high density lipoproteins.** *Circulation* 1979, **60**:1220–1229.
Randomized trial of exercise plus dietary advice versus dietary advice alone in over 100 Finnish men aged 40–45, which examined changes in lipoprotein cholesterol and HDL apoproteins.

11

12 DRUG TREATMENT OF HYPERLIPIDAEMIA

Introduction

Lipid-lowering drugs should always be used as an adjunct to dietary measures rather than as an alternative. Most well motivated people with mild-to-moderate hyperlipidaemia respond to diet alone but severe cases may be more resistant. Detailed criteria upon which decisions on the need for drug therapy should be based are dealt with in the final chapter.

In general terms, the use of lipid-lowering drugs should be reserved for individuals at high risk for CHD or with severe hypercholesterolaemia who do not respond adequately to diet, whereas drug therapy is often used as an adjunct to diet in the context of secondary intervention.

12

There are various ways in which lipid-lowering drugs can be classified; perhaps the most useful from the clinician's viewpoint is to subdivide them according to whether their predominant effect is on triglyceride-rich or cholesterol-rich lipoproteins. Obviously there will be some overlap in the spectrum of drug effects, just as there is overlap between the different types of hyperlipidaemia.

Triglyceride-lowering drugs

There are three main classes of triglyceride-lowering agents: fibrates, nicotinic acid compounds and the fish-oil preparations such as Maxepa® (ω3 marine triglycerides, Glaxo). The chief quantitative change achieved by all three classes is a reduction in VLDL levels. LDL cholesterol levels are reduced by nicotinic acid compounds whereas the fibrates and Maxepa may increase or decrease LDL, depending upon the type of hyperlipidaemia being treated. These drugs are mainly used in the treatment of types IIb, III, IV and V hyperlipoproteinaemia. However, since they often induce a desirable increase in HDL cholesterol, this also makes them potentially useful adjuncts to cholesterol-lowering drugs with a predominant effect on LDL cholesterol (*see* Combination Drug Therapy).

Fibrates
Clofibrate
Clofibrate [2-(p-chlorphenoxy)-2-methyl propionate] has been used to treat hyperlipidaemia for the past 25 years but is gradually becoming obsolete. This is in part due to its now well established lithogenic side effects and in part to the emergence of more potent and safer fibrates. However, since it is the prototype of its class its properties will be dealt with in some detail.

Clofibrate has several pharmacological actions, which include stimulation of lipolysis by increasing adipose tissue-derived lipoprotein lipase. In plasma over 98% is bound to albumin and its half-life in the body is 12 hours, excretion being almost entirely via the kidney as the glucuronide. Concurrent administration of cholestyramine does not impair its absorption.

Daily doses of 0.5–1 g twice daily result in a 15–20% decrease in serum total cholesterol and a 30–40% decrease in serum triglyceride [1]. These effects are most prominent in patients with type III or type IV hyperlipidaemia. Turnover studies show that clofibrate stimulates VLDL catabolism without altering its rate of synthesis. This effect is often accompanied in type IV hyperlipoproteinaemia by an undesirable increase in LDL cholesterol, which is partially offset by a potentially beneficial increase in HDL cholesterol. Patients with type III hyperlipoproteinaemia often respond dramatically with virtual normalization of serum lipids and regression of cutaneous xanthomata (Fig. 12.1). This is probably the only remaining indication for clofibrate.

Mobilization of tissue cholesterol by clofibrate is accompanied by an increase in biliary cholesterol secretion and faecal neutral steroid excretion. The increased cholesterol content of bile was responsible for a twofold increase in the incidence of gallstones in the WHO trial and the Coronary Drug Project, the mortality associated with gall-bladder disease being a major contributory factor to the excess of deaths from non-cardiovascular disease observed in the WHO trial [2].

12

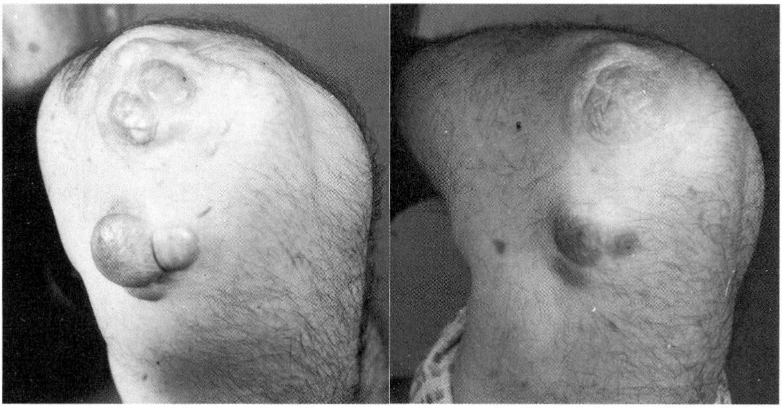

Fig. 12.1. Regression of tubero-eruptive xanthomata in type III hyperlipoproteinaemia after 33 months' treatment with diet and clofibrate 2 g daily.

Apart from gallstones the other major side effect of clofibrate is an acute myalgic or myositic syndrome characterized by pain in the thighs or calves and by an increase in CPK. Patients with renal impairment or the nephrotic syndrome are particularly prone to this complication, which rapidly resolves once the drug is withdrawn. Clofibrate enhances the effect of anti-coagulants, the dosage of which should be halved initially, and hypoglycaemia may occur if clofibrate is given with the sulphonylureas in diabetics.

Bezafibrate
Bezafibrate (2-[4-[2-(4-chlorobenzamido)ethyl]phenoxy]-2-methyl-propionic acid) is more potent than clofibrate in reducing serum cholesterol and triglycerides. The precise mechanism is unknown but may include inhibition of the enzyme acetyl-CoA carboxylase on the fatty acid synthesis pathway. Like clofibrate it increases the activity of adipose tissue lipoprotein lipase but it differs in also increasing the activity of hepatic lipase and in having a shorter half-life in plasma.

A comparison between clofibrate and bezafibrate showed that the latter decreased serum and VLDL triglyceride levels more effectively in type IV hyperlipoproteinaemia but there was little difference between them in lowering LDL cholesterol and raising HDL cholesterol levels in type IIa or IIb hyperlipoproteinaemia [3]. Serum triglycerides markedly decreased in those with type IV and IIb phenotypes on bezafibrate but a significant rise in LDL cholesterol has been observed in type IV patients. However, in hypercholesterolaemic subjects bezafibrate reduces LDL levels by stimulating receptor-mediated FCR, although this effect is to some extent offset by increased conversion of VLDL to LDL [4]. The drug was well tolerated over a period of 6 months when

12

administered to children with FH and lowered total cholesterol by 22% [5]. Other reported actions of bezafibrate include improvement of glucose tolerance in hypertriglyceridaemic patients and reduction of plasma viscosity.

The recommended dosage is 200 mg thrice daily but a daily dose of the long-acting preparation Bezalip-Mono 400 mg is claimed to be just as effective.

The half-life of the drug in plasma is prolonged and its concentration is increased in patients with renal failure which may necessitate decreasing the dose. Gastrointestinal side effects, especially nausea and distension, are not uncommon and impotence and a myositic syndrome similar to that seen with clofibrate have also been described. So far there is no evidence of an increased incidence of gallstones in patients taking the drug but this remains a definite possibility.

Gemfibrozil
Gemfibrozil (5-(2,5-dimethylphenoxy)-2,2-dimethyl-pentanoic acid) is a homologue of clofibrate but unlike the latter and bezafibrate it is not halogenated, which may be advantageous with respect to long-term toxicity. Its mechanism of action is similar to other fibrates but it reduces triglycerides to a greater extent [6], although it decreases LDL cholesterol less than bezafibrate [7]. It appears to be less prone to cause lithogenic side effects than clofibrate as judged from the results of the Helsinki Heart Study [8], but it causes a similar increase in biliary cholesterol excretion.

Over the 5 years of that trial, the average changes in serum lipids induced by gemfibrozil 600 mg twice daily were an 11% decrease in total cholesterol, 10% decrease of LDL cholesterol, 43% decrease in triglyceride and a 10% increase in HDL cholesterol [9]. When these changes were analysed according to lipoprotein phenotype the decreases in LDL cholesterol were greater in type IIa than in type IIb whereas a rise occurred in type IV patients. Reductions in triglyceride were greatest in type IV patients whereas rises in HDL cholesterol were similar in all three groups (Fig. 12.2). As discussed in the final chapter these changes were accompanied by a significant decrease in the incidence of CHD as compared with placebo-treated controls. Statistical analysis suggested that the beneficial effects of gemfibrozil were due partly to the reduction in LDL cholesterol and partly to the increase in HDL cholesterol but, surprisingly, not to the reduction in triglyceride, which in percentage terms showed the greatest change.

Gemfibrozil has an even shorter half-life than bezafibrate but is metabolized in a similar manner. Adverse effects are similar to those observed with the other fibrates, gastrointestinal upset being the commonest.

Other fibrates
Other fibrates which appear to be more potent in their LDL-lowering effects than any of those mentioned so far are ciprofibrate and fenofibrate [7]. The availability of the different fibrates varies in Europe, North America and Australasia, with gemfibrozil, clofibrate and bezafibrate being the most widely

12

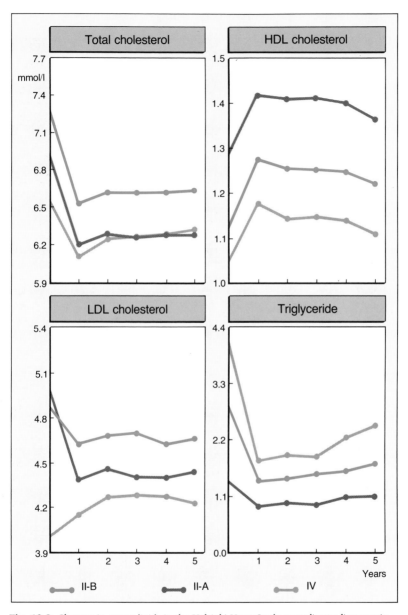

Fig. 12.2. Changes in serum lipids in the Helsinki Heart Study according to lipoprotein phenotype during administration of gemfibrozil 1.2 g daily. Adapted by permission [9].

12

available. However, fenofibrate is widely used in France and has the advantage of also lowering uric acid levels.

Nicotinic acid compounds

Nicotinic acid would be more widely used were it not for its side effects. Like the fibrates it reduces both cholesterol and triglyceride but especially the latter, decreases of 10 and 28%, respectively, being observed on a dose of 3 g per day in the Coronary Drug Project [10]. These changes are due to decreases in VLDL synthesis but without the enhanced conversion of VLDL into LDL which occurs in type IV patients on fibrates. Decreased synthesis of VLDL is secondary to reduced influx of FFA from adipose tissue, reflecting the anti-lipolytic action of the drug, and results in a fall in LDL cholesterol.

Another important action of nicotinic acid is to raise HDL cholesterol, especially HDL_2. Studies of apoA-I turnover suggest that this effect is due to a drug-induced decrease in HDL catabolism.

The most prominent side effect of nicotinic acid, and its compounds or analogues, is cutaneous vasodilatation. This is maximal during the first weeks of therapy but thereafter a degree of tolerance develops, especially if the dose is increased gradually from 0.25 g once to thrice daily to a maximum of 1–2 g thrice daily. Aspirin given beforehand helps minimize nicotinic acid-induced flushing and the drug should always be taken with or after a meal. Hot drinks may exacerbate the flushing. Other adverse effects are skin rashes, gastrointestinal upsets, hyperuricaemia, hyperglycaemia and hepatic dysfunction. There was also an increased incidence of arrhythmias in the nicotinic acid group during the Coronary Drug Project.

Despite the problems associated with the taking of effective doses of nicotinic acid, there is increasing evidence from both primary and secondary prevention trials that administration of this drug on a long-term basis, either alone or in conjunction with a fibrate, leads to a reduction in both coronary and total mortality. Another advantage is its ability to potentiate a neomycin-induced decrease of Lp(a) levels, at the same time offsetting the decrease in HDL cholesterol induced by the latter drug [11].

12

Various preparations are available, including nicofuranose and acipimox. The latter is 5-methylpyrazine carboxylic acid 4-oxide and in a dose of 750–1200 mg/day has been shown to decrease serum triglyceride and increase HDL cholesterol in patients with type IV and type V hyperlipoproteinaemia [12]. Unlike the fibrates it does not increase post-heparin lipolytic activity but hepatic lipase activity is reduced, which may explain the rise in HDL_2 which occurs. The drug is not protein bound, has a half-life of 2 hours, and is excreted unchanged in the urine. Nicotinamide, widely available in health-food shops, is ineffective as a lipid-lowering agent.

Fish-oil

It had long been known that Greenland Eskimos have much lower plasma triglyceride levels than their Danish compatriots. Subsequent studies showed that this effect can be reproduced in non-Eskimos by feeding them oil derived from the bodies of fatty fish, rich in the long-chain, highly polyunsaturated ω3 fatty acids eicosapentaenoic acid (EPA) and docosahexaenoic acid (DHA). Phillipson *et al.* [13] treated 20 hypertriglyceridaemic patients with a diet in which 20–30% of the calories were provided by salmon-oil or a commercially available preparation (Maxepa). Ten patients had type IIb hyperlipoproteinaemia; the other 10 had type V hyperlipoproteinaemia. When compared with conventional low-fat or modified-fat diets the fish-oil diet decreased plasma total cholesterol and triglyceride by 27 and 64%, respectively, in the type IIb patients and by 45 and 79% in the type V patients (Fig. 12.3). These changes were due to marked decreases in VLDL in type IIb subjects and chylomicrons in type V subjects.

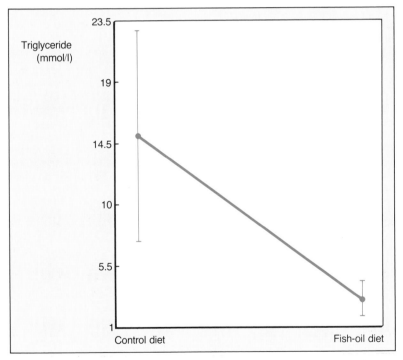

Fig. 12.3. Changes in levels of plasma triglyceride (mean ± s.d.) in 10 patients with the type V phenotype on fish oil. Adapted by permission [13].

Administration of a lower dose of Maxepa (15 g/day) to 20 hypertriglyceridaemic men confirmed the triglyceride-lowering effect of the fish-oil preparation. The amounts of EPA and DHA provided by the Maxepa were 2.7 g and 1.9 g, respectively, equivalent to consuming 200–250 g of fatty fish. Turnover studies showed that the decrease in plasma triglyceride was due to a marked reduction in VLDL triglyceride synthesis [14]. This finding is in accord with other evidence that fish-oil decreases the rate of synthesis of VLDL-apoB. However, the triglyceride-lowering effect of this dose of Maxepa was accompanied by a rise in LDL-apoB levels, possibly due to changes in VLDL particle size which lead to increased conversion of VLDL to LDL (Table 12.1).

Table 12.1. Effect of Maxepa 15 g/day on serum total cholesterol (TC), triglyceride (TG) and LDL-apoB levels in patients with hypertriglyceridaemia (mean ± s.d.)

Period	n	TC (mmol/l)	TG (mmol/l)	LDL apoB (mg/dl)
Pre-Maxepa	23	6.9 ± 4.7	6.9 ± 8.5	112 ± 41
2 weeks	16	6.5 ± 4.8	3.0 ± 3.3*	131 ± 50*
4 weeks	23	6.8 ± 4.4	3.6 ± 3.3*	125 ± 40*
8 weeks	11	6.9 ± 4.7	3.6 ± 3.50*	125 ± 51
Post-Maxepa†	12	6.2 ± 5.3	6.5 ± 5.9	114 ± 31

*$P < 0.05$ versus pre-Maxepa values. †4 weeks after discontinuation. Published by permission from Sullivan et al., Atherosclerosis 1986, 61:129–134.

The ability of high doses of Maxepa to reduce triglyceride synthesis in type V hyperlipoproteinaemia is an undoubted asset but the tendency of moderate doses (10–15 g/day) to increase LDL levels in type IV patients is potentially deleterious. However, it is possible that this is offset by other, more beneficial effects, which include alterations in platelet function and prostaglandin formation, reductions in plasma fibrinogen, and decreased generation of leukotrienes by monocytes, as reviewed elsewhere [14]. These effects may have a bearing on recent reports that administration of fish-oil reduces the rate of restenosis after angioplasty, although this remains to be confirmed. The opposite has also been claimed, namely that auto-oxidation of these highly polyunsaturated fatty acids occurs *in vivo* and promotes atherosclerosis. Thus although they have an important albeit limited use in the management of type V hyperlipoproteinaemia their role in preventing atherosclerosis remains unproven, despite the epidemiological evidence in its favour. They are ineffective in treating primary hypercholesterolaemia unless given in extremely high doses.

12

Cholesterol-lowering drugs

These drugs act chiefly by reducing LDL cholesterol. In some instances this is accompanied by a concomitant decrease in HDL cholesterol whereas in others HDL cholesterol levels tend to rise, depending upon the drug used. Likewise triglyceride levels may change in either direction, again depending upon the choice of drug. Cholesterol-lowering drugs are either used singly or in combination to treat type IIa hyperlipoproteinaemia, especially if due to FH, or together with a triglyceride-lowering drug to treat type IIb hyperlipoproteinaemia, especially if due to FCH.

Anion-exchange resins

The anion-exchange resins used to treat hypercholesterolaemia are insoluble compounds which act by binding bile acids within the intestinal lumen, thus interfering with their reabsorption and enhancing their faecal excretion. As a result bile acid synthesis is markedly stimulated and this results in an increased requirement for cholesterol in the liver, which is partly met by up-regulation of hepatic LDL receptors and an increased rate of removal of LDL from plasma. The consequent reduction in LDL cholesterol makes these drugs especially useful in the treatment of heterozygous FH, where LDL levels are high because of a partial defect of receptor-mediated LDL catabolism. However, their effectiveness is constrained by their unpalatability. They are ineffective in homozygotes.

Cholestyramine

Cholestyramine, a polymer containing quaternary ammonium groups, exchanges chloride ions for bile acid anions within the intestinal lumen. It comes as a powder which must be suspended in liquid before ingestion. It is given in doses of 8–24 g per day, usually in two or three divided doses, but many patients find it difficult to ingest more than two sachets (each 9 g sachet containing 4 g resin) twice daily on account of the gastrointestinal side effects of the drug.

Cholestyramine has been in use for over 20 years and has been tested extensively. In the LRC Primary Prevention Trial almost 2000 men with moderate type IIa or IIb hyperlipoproteinaemia, mainly non-FH, were given 24 g per day for over 7 years. During this time their mean total cholesterol was 8.5% lower, LDL cholesterol 12.6% lower, HDL cholesterol 3% higher and triglyceride 4.5% higher than placebo-treated controls [15]. However, almost 30% of patients discontinued taking the drug before the end of the trial. Much greater reductions in total and LDL cholesterol were observed in subjects known to be taking at least 20 g per day throughout although it is of interest that even in this group the reduction of LDL cholesterol was less at 7 years (26%) than at 1 year (33%). This lessening of effect with time together with its tendency to induce hypertriglyceridaemia reflects the compensatory increase in VLDL synthesis which the drug engenders, making it unsuitable for patients with hypertriglyceridaemia. Similar results were obtained in the NHLBI type II Coronary Intervention Study in patients with severe hypercholesterolaemia, many of whom had FH, as illustrated in Fig. 12.4.

12

The most frequent side effects are constipation, which occasionally leads to intestinal obstruction, and a tendency to aggravate or cause indigestion. Be-

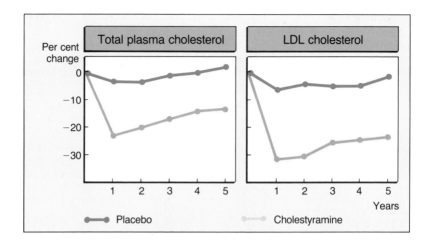

Fig. 12.4. Mean per cent change in total plasma cholesterol and LDL cholesterol achieved by cholestyramine in type II patients. Adapted by permission from Levy *et al.*, *Circulation* 1984, 69:325–337.

cause it interferes with the absorption of iron and folic acid, oral supplements of both should be given to children taking the drug. Impaired absorption of digoxin and thyroxine can also present a problem unless these drugs are administered between doses of cholestyramine.

Colestipol hydrochloride
Colestipol, a co-polymer of tetraethylenepentamine and epichlorhydrin, has a similar mode of action to cholestyramine. The usual daily dose in adults is two 5 g sachets twice daily. Apart from cholestyramine, it is probably the only safe drug to use in the treatment of hypercholesterolaemic children. There is little to choose between cholestyramine and colestipol with regard to extent of LDL lowering achieved and adverse effects are similar, including aggravation of hypertriglyceridaemia and gastrointestinal disturbances [16]. However, some patients find it easier to take than its longer-established rival. The fact that neither drug is absorbed renders the likelihood of serious systemic side effects remote and is reassuring to patient and physician alike.

Neomycin
This poorly absorbed antibiotic is an effective cholesterol-lowering agent when given in doses of 0.5–1.0 g twice daily. Long-term administration results in a decrease in serum cholesterol of up to 30% in patients with FH, which is comparable to the effect achieved by 16 g of cholestyramine per day. Neomycin acts by precipitating cholesterol within the intestinal lumen and thus

inhibiting its absorption. This effect is the result of interaction between the cationic groups of the aminoglucoside and the anionic components of the mixed micelles within which cholesterol is solubilized. In some studies this has led to a reduction in LDL cholesterol and not in HDL cholesterol [17] but in others HDL cholesterol levels decreased. Side effects include nausea, which can be offset by taking the drug with food, and diarrhoea. In the long term neomycin can cause ototoxicity but this complication seldom occurs in the absence of impaired renal function. Usefulness of the drug has been limited by worries about adverse effects during long-term administration and by the high frequencey of diarrhoea, although recent observations that it can lower Lp(a) levels may give it a new lease of life [11].

Probucol

Probucol (4,4-(isopropylidenedithio)bis(2,b-di-t-butylphenol)) is a moderately effective cholesterol-lowering agent which has little effect on serum triglyceride. When given in a dose of 0.5 g twice daily it reduced serum cholesterol by 20% and 12% in patients with type IIa or IIb and type IV phenotypes, respectively. Reductions in serum cholesterol of around 10% have been observed in FH patients. The decrease in serum cholesterol reflects falls in both LDL cholesterol and HDL cholesterol but the mechanisms involved are unclear. Interestingly the fall in LDL cholesterol induced by probucol is greater in FH patients with the $\varepsilon 4$ allele than in those with the normal apoE$_3$/E$_3$ phenotype [18]. Despite reducing HDL cholesterol probucol causes regression of xanthelasma, the latter effect being greatest in patients showing the most marked decrease in HDL cholesterol. This is of considerable interest in that it implies that a low HDL cholesterol is not necessarily disadvantageous. Additional evidence that the anti-oxidant properties of probucol prevent lipid peroxidation, thereby inhibiting LDL uptake by macrophages and reducing atherogenesis in experimental animals [19], suggests that the drug may have beneficial effects that have little to do with its LDL-lowering properties, although this remains to be confirmed in humans.

HMG CoA reductase inhibitors

These drugs act by competitively inhibiting HMG CoA reductase and thereby block conversion of HMG CoA into mevalonic acid. They are very potent inhibitors of the enzyme with K_1 values in the range 0.2–2.2×10^{-9} M compared with the K_m of the substrate, which is 4×10^{-6} M. As a result, cholesterol synthesis is inhibited, especially in the liver which requires cholesterol as a substrate for bile acid synthesis. To overcome the short-fall, hepatocytes express a greater number of LDL receptors and thereby promote influx of LDL cholesterol from plasma. The net result is a dose-dependent decrease in plasma cholesterol. As might be expected these drugs are relatively ineffective in patients with homozygous FH, who lack LDL receptors, but they work well in heterozygotes, who have only a partial deficiency.

12

The first HMG CoA reductase inhibitor to be developed was compactin, a fungal metabolite, now called mevastatin. Lovastatin, originally called mevinolin, was isolated simultaneously but independently by Endo and Alberts from different moulds [20] and differs from mevastatin only in having an additional methyl group. Simvastatin, previously called synvinolin, is very similar to lovastatin but possesses an extra methyl group in the side chain, inserted synthetically. A fourth compound, which is a derivative of mevastatin, is pravastatin, previously known as eptastatin. Simvastatin is a more potent inhibitor of HMG CoA reductase than lovastatin which, in turn, is more potent than pravastatin. The latter remains an investigational drug but both lovastatin and simvastatin have been approved for use in many countries.

Lovastatin and simvastatin are both lactones and are inactive until metabolized in the liver to the open ring hydroxy acids. In contrast pravastatin is a hydroxy acid. It has been suggested that because of these differences the level of lovastatin and simvastatin in blood and non-hepatic tissues is lower than that of pravastatin, relative to their concentrations in the liver.

These drugs have a similar spectrum of action to the anion-exchange resins: namely, they primarily lower LDL cholesterol, but are more potent and better tolerated. Also at high doses they reduce serum triglycerides to some extent whereas anion-exchange resins do the opposite. Both types of drugs induce a small increase in HDL cholesterol but neither has any effect in reducing Lp(a) levels. HMG CoA reductase inhibitors are more effective than anion-exchange resins and probucol in lowering LDL cholesterol (Table 12.2) but they are less effective than the fibrates in reducing serum triglycerides and in raising HDL cholesterol [21].

Table 12.2. Comparison of lovastatin, cholestyramine, gemfibrozil and probucol in hypercholesterolaemic patients treated for 12–14 weeks.

Daily dose	Mean percentage change			
	TC	LDL-C	HDL-C	TG
Cholestyramine 24 g*	− 17%	− 23%	+ 8%	+ 11%
Probucol 1 g*	− 9%	− 9%	− 23%	+ 3%
Lovastatin 40 mg†	− 28%	− 35%	+ 6%	− 12%
Gemfibrozil 1.2 g†	− 16%	− 18%	+ 12%	− 40%

*Henwood and Heel, *Drugs* 1988, 36:429–454; †[21].

Both lovastatin and simvastatin are very easy to take, the former being given in doses of 20–80 mg in a once- or twice-daily regimen, the latter in doses of 10–40 mg once daily in the evening, so as to offset the nocturnal in ease in HMG CoA reductase activity and cholesterol synthesis. These drugs are particularly effective in reducing LDL cholesterol in heterozygous FH, as shown in Table 12.3. They are also useful in treating polygenic hypercholesterolaemia, as illustrated in Fig. 12.5, and in treating patients with hypercholesterolaemia secondary to the nephrotic syndrome [22].

Table 12.3. Comparative effects of HMG CoA reductase inhibitors in patients with heterozygous FH.

Dose (mg)	Decrease in LDL cholesterol (%)		
	Lovastatin	Simvastatin	Pravastatin
10	20	28	2
20	26	36	31
40	33	41	–
80	39	46	–

Data calculated from [7].

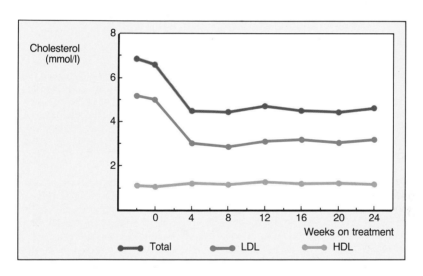

Fig. 12.5. Effect of simvastatin 20 mg/day on total, LDL and HDL cholesterol concentrations (mean ± s.e.m., n = 10) in patients with polygenic hypercholesterolaemia. Adapted by permission from Mölgaard *et al, Eur Heart J* 1988, 9:541–551.

12

Greatest experience to date has been obtained with lovastatin, which has been licensed for use in the USA for two years and administered to patients on a compassionate-use basis for over 5 years [23]. Turnover studies have shown that this drug stimulates receptor-mediated LDL catabolism in FH heterozygotes and decreases both VLDL and LDL synthesis in polygenic hypercholesterolaemia. The main side effect has been a reversible myositic syndrome in roughly 0.5% of patients; this was severe enough to cause rhab-domyolysis and transient renal failure in at least three cardiac transplant patients on cyclosporine. HMG CoA reductase inhibitors should be used with great caution in such patients and in those with hepatic dysfunction. The risk of myositis is also greater when these drugs are used in conjunction with fibrates and nicotinic acid. Although there is no evidence that they impair steroid synthesis in the adrenal cortex or gonads their use is not advised in children or in women who might become pregnant. Anxieties that they might cause cataracts in man appear to be unfounded [24].

This new class of drug has already revolutionized the management of severe hypercholesterolaemia, especially FH, and it is possible that alone or in combination with other lipid-lowering measures they may eventually have as profound an effect on atherosclerosis as had penicillin, another fungal metabolite, on infectious disease.

Combination drug therapy

Often combinations of two lipid-lowering drugs control hyperlipidaemia better than either drug given alone. There are several reasons for using combination drug therapy: (1) to treat mixed hyperlipidaemias; (2) to offset undesirable changes in serum lipids which may accompany single drug therapy; (3) to achieve a synergistic effect in refractory cases of severe hyperlipidaemia; (4) to increase the cost-effectiveness of therapy, by using low doses of two drugs rather than high doses of one.

The first two categories of usage are exemplified by the combined use of gem-fibrozil and either colestipol or lovastatin to treat patients with FCH [25]. In those with type IIb phenotypes gemfibrozil reduced triglycerides and raised HDL cholesterol but did not reduce LDL cholesterol. Addition of colestipol or lovastatin achieved the latter effect. In the type IV patients gemfibrozil again reduced triglycerides and raised HDL cholesterol but increased LDL cholesterol by 29%, whereas addition of either colestipol or lovastatin reduced LDL cholesterol by over 30%. Overall the best results were obtained by gemfibrozil plus lovastatin, although this combination should be used cautiously in view of the increased frequency of myositic complications [24]. Combination of a fibric acid derivative and lovastatin has also been used to good effect in type III hyperlipoproteinaemia [7].

The third use of combination drug therapy, namely to maximize the extent of lipid-lowering achievable, applies particularly to patients with FH. Some of the various combinations which have been used and a comparison of the decreases in LDL cholesterol obtained are shown in Table 12.4. Note the more than 60% reduction achieved by the formidable combination of colestipol (30 g), nicotinic acid (1.5–7.5 g) and lovastatin (40–60 mg). Almost as great reductions of LDL can be obtained with the more acceptable combination of

12

lovastatin 40 mg and cholestyramine 4–8 g each given twice daily [7], although increases in HDL cholesterol are probably less marked without nicotinic acid. The triple-drug combination was also reported to reduce LDL cholesterol by almost 60% in an FH homozygote, which is remarkable [26]. Patients requiring combination drug therapy are best managed in a specialized lipid clinic.

Table 12.4. Effect of combination drug therapy on LDL cholesterol in patients with heterozygous FH.

Combination		LDL cholesterol (mmol/l, pre-therapy)	% Decrease
Resin*	+ bezafibrate	6.7–7.2[†]	31–39[†]
	+ probucol	7.7–8.9	32–53
	+ nicotinic acid	6.8–9.6	32–55
Lovastatin	+ probucol	8.9	42
	+ resin	8.3–10.2	52–54
	+ nicotinic acid	8.4–9.9	49–55
	+ resin + nicotinic acid	8.4–9.6	62–67

*Cholestyramine or colestipol. Adapted by permission from [7]. [†]From Curtis et al., Br Med J 1988, 297:173–175.

Annotated references

1.   OLIVER MF: **The present status of clofibrate (Atromid-S).** *Circulation* 1967, 36:337–339.
Editorial summarizing experience with the drug in the hopeful era before the WHO trial.

2.   REPORT FROM THE COMMITTEE OF PRINCIPAL INVESTIGATORS: **A co-operative trial in the primary prevention of ischaemic heart disease using clofibrate.** *Br Heart J* 1978, 40:1069–1118.
Disappointing results of the WHO trial which showed 25% more deaths in the clofibrate group than in the high cholesterol controls.

3.   OLLSON A, ROSSNER S, WALLDIUS G, CARLSON LA, LANG PD: **Effect of BM 15.075 on lipoprotein concentrations in different types of hyperlipoproteinaemia.** *Atherosclerosis* 1977, 27:279–287.
Swedish comparison of lipid-lowering effects of two fibrates.

4.   STEWART JM, PACKARD CJ, LORIMER AR, BOAG DE, SHEPHERD J: **Effects of bezafibrate on receptor-mediated and receptor-independent low density lipoprotein catabolism in type II hyperlipoproteinaemic subjects.** *Atherosclerosis* 1982, 44:355–365.
Results of LDL turnover studies in seven hypercholesterolaemic subjects before and during bezafibrate therapy.

12

5.   WHEELER KAH, WEST RJ, LLOYD JK, BARLEY J: **Double blind trial of bezafibrate in familial hypercholesterolaemia.** *Arch Dis Child* 1985, 60:34–37.

Controlled trial of bezafibrate in children with familial hypercholesterolaemia with encouraging results.

6.   KESANIEMI YA, GRUNDY SM: **Influence of gemfibrozil and clofibrate on metabolism of cholesterol and plasma triglycerides in man.** *JAMA* 1984, 251:2241–2246.

Comparative study of effects of clofibrate and gemfibrozil on VLDL triglyceride turnover and cholesterol balance.

7.   ILLINGWORTH DR: **Drug therapy of hypercholesterolemia.** *Clin Chem* 1988, 34:B123–B132.

Up-to-date and comprehensive review article.

8.   FRICK MH, ELO O, HAAPA K, HEINONEN OP, HEINSALMI P, HELO P, HUTTUNEN JK, KAITANIEMI P, KOSKINEN P, MANNINEN V, MAENPAA H, MALKONEN M, MANTAARI M, NOROLA S, PASTERNACK A, PIKKARAINEN J, ROMO M, SJOBLOM T, NIKKILA EA: **Helsinki Heart Study: Primary prevention trial with gemfibrozil in middle-aged men with dyslipidaemia.** *N Engl J Med* 1987, 317:1237–1245.

First description of the beneficial outcome of the Helsinki Heart Study and lesser incidence of adverse effects compared with the WHO clofibrate trial.

9.   MANNINEN V, ELO MO, FRICK MH, HAAPA K, HEINONEN OP, HEINSALMI P, HELO P, HUTTUNEN JK, KAITANIEMI P, KOSKINEN P, MAENPAA H, MALKONEN M, MANTAARI M, NOROLA S, PASTERNACK A, PIKKARAINEN J, ROMO M, SJOBLOM T, NIKKILA EA: **Lipid alterations and decline in the incidence of coronary heart disease in the Helsinki Heart Study.** *JAMA* 1988, 260:641–651.

Further analysis of the results of the Helsinki Heart Study broken down according to phenotype.

10.   CORONARY DRUG PROJECT RESEARCH GROUP: **Clofibrate and niacin in coronary heart disease.** *JAMA* 1975, 231:360–381.

Initially disappointing results of the Coronary Drug Project.

11.   GURAKAR A, HOEG JM, KOSTNER G, PAPADOPOULOS NM, BREWER HB: **Levels of lipoprotein Lp(a) decline with neomycin and niacin treatment.** *Atherosclerosis* 1985, 57:293–301.

Neomycin and nicotinic acid seem to be the only two drugs reported so far to reduce Lp(a) levels.

12.   TASKINEN M-R, NIKKILA EA: **Effects of acipimox on serum lipids, lipoproteins and lipolytic enzymes in hypertriglyceridemia.** *Atherosclerosis* 1988, 69:249–255.

Description of a new nicotinic acid analogue.

13.   PHILLIPSON BE, ROTHROCK DW, CONNOR WE, HARRIS WS, ILLINGWORTH DR: **Reduction of plasma lipids, lipoproteins, and apoproteins by dietary fish oils in patients with hypertriglyceridemia.** *N Engl J Med* 1985, 312:1210–1216.

First description of the remarkable effectiveness of fish-oil in the treatment of severe hypertriglyceridaemia.

12

14. THOMPSON GR: **Lipids, fish and coronary heart disease.** *Curr Opin Cardiol* 1986, 1:827–831.
Review article of the multiplicity of actions whereby fish oil may influence atherosclerosis.

15. LIPID RESEARCH CLINICS PROGRAM: **The Lipid Research Clinics Coronary Primary Prevention Trial results. I. Reduction in incidence of coronary heart disease.** *JAMA* 1984, **251**:351–364.
Description of effects of long-term cholestyramine administration including side effects.

16. GLUECK CJ, FORD S, SCHEEL D, STEINER P: **Colestipol and cholestyramine resin. Comparative effects in familial type II hyperlipoproteinemia.** *JAMA* 1972, **222**:676–681.
Comparison of two anion-exchange resins in 25 type II patients.

17. HOEG JM, SCHAEFER EJ, ROMANO CA, BON E, PIKUS AM, ZECH LA, BAILEY KR, GREGG RE, WILSON PWF, SPRECHER DL, GRIMES AM, SEBRING NG, AYRES EJ, JAHN CE, BREWER HB: **Neomycin and plasma lipoproteins in type II hyperlipoproteinemia.** *Clin Pharmacol Ther* 1984, **36**:555–565.
Double-blind trial of neomycin versus placebo in 20 type II patients.

18. NESTRUCK AC, BOUTHILLIER D, SING CF, DAVIGNON J: **Apolipoprotein E polymorphism and plasma cholesterol response to probucol.** *Metabolism* 1987, **36**:743–747.
Intriguing observation on the relation between apoE phenotype and the cholesterol-lowering effect of probucol.

19. KITA T, NAGANO Y, YOKODE M, ISHII K, OOSHIMA A, YOSHIDA H, KAWAI C: **Probucol prevents the progression of atherosclerosis in Watanabe heritable hyperlipidemic rabbit, an animal model for familial hypercholesterolemia.** *Proc Natl Acad Sci USA* 1987, **84**:5928–5931.
Important observation that the anti-atherogenic effect of probucol in Watanabe rabbits may be due to its anti-oxidant properties.

20. ALBERTS AW: **HMG-CoA reductase inhibitors — the development.** *Atherosclerosis Rev* 1988, **18**:123–131.
Useful review of the mode of action of HMG CoA reductase inhibitors by one of the discoverers of lovastatin.

21. TIKKANEN MJ, HELVE E, JÄÄTTELÄ, KAARSALO E, LEHTONEN A, MALBECQ W, OKSA H, PÄÄKKÖNEN P, SALMI J, VEHARANTA T, VIIKARI J, ÄÄRYNEN M: **Comparison between lovastatin and gemfibrozil in the treatment of primary hypercholesterolemia: the Finnish multicenter study.** *Am J Cardiol* 1988, **62**:35J–43J.
Double-blind comparison of lovastatin and gemfibrozil in patients with moderate hypercholesterolaemia with or without moderate hypertriglyceridaemia.

22. RABELINK AJ, HENE RH, ERKELENS DW, JOLES JA, KOOMANS HA: **Effects of simvastatin and cholestyramine on lipoprotein profile in hyperlipidaemia of nephrotic syndrome.** *Lancet* 1988, **ii**:1335–1338.
Superiority of simvastatin over cholestyramine in lowering LDL cholesterol was demonstrated in 10 patients with the nephrotic syndrome.

12

23.   ILLINGWORTH DR, BACON SP, LARSEN KK: **Long-term experience with HMG-CoA reductase inhibitors in the therapy of hypercholesterolemia.** *Atherosclerosis Rev* 1988, **18**:161–187.
Detailed account of the authors' considerable experience of using lovastatin and simvastatin.

24.   TOBERT JA: **Efficacy and long-term adverse effect pattern of lovastatin.** *Am J Cardiol* 1988, **62**:28J–34J.
Review of the pros and cons of lovastatin through the eyes of a physician who was intimately involved in the clinical trials of this compound.

25.   EAST C, BILHEIMER DW, GRUNDY SM: **Combination drug therapy for familial combined hyperlipidemia.** *Ann Intern Med* 1988, **109**:25–32.
Description of the synergistic effects of lovastatin and gemfibrozil in familial combined hyperlipidaemia.

26.   MALLOY MJ, KANE JP, KUNITAKE ST, TUN P: **Complementarity of colestipol, niacin, and lovastatin in treatment of severe familial hypercholesterolemia.** *Ann Intern Med* 1987, **107**:616–623.
Remarkable reductions in LDL cholesterol and apoB and increases in HDL cholesterol and apoA-I achieved by triple-drug therapy in 22 patients with FH.

12

13 RADICAL THERAPY FOR REFRACTORY HYPERLIPIDAEMIA

Introduction
Extracorporeal removal of lipoproteins
Plasma exchange
LDL apheresis
Other techniques

Surgical procedures
Partial ileal bypass
Portacaval shunt
Liver transplantation

Gene replacement therapy
Annotated references

Introduction

Radical, or non-pharmacological, methods of treatment should never be used until it has first been shown that conventional therapy either fails to control hyperlipidaemia or cannot be tolerated by the patient. Such methods include the surgical procedures of partial ileal bypass, portacaval shunt and liver transplantation, and medical manoeuvres such as plasma exchange and LDL apheresis. In general the use of these techniques will be restricted to patients with severe FH, although occasionally they may be resorted to in other categories of hyperlipidaemia, as discussed below.

Extracorporeal removal of lipoproteins

The first attempt to treat hypercholesterolaemia by extracorporeal means was undertaken in 1965 by De Gennes and colleagues, who performed manual plasmapheresis repetitively in a patient with homozygous FH. However, this approach was too tedious for prolonged use and was soon abandoned.

In that same year a development occurred that subsequently revolutionized the field — the introduction of the continuous flow blood cell separator. Used initially for leukopheresis, the first plasma exchanges with this machine for hypercholesterolaemia were performed in 1972 to treat a patient with xanthomatous neuropathy complicating primary biliary cirrhosis [1]. Other more recent approaches include the techniques of LDL apheresis and double filtration plasmapheresis, both of which are intended to remove selectively LDL cholesterol rather than the entire spectrum of lipoprotein particles, as is achieved by plasma exchange. Although there are theoretical reasons why selectivity can be useful when treating FH the non-selectivity of plasma exchange can be useful in other circumstances, especially when treating severe hypertriglyceridaemia.

Plasma exchange

Plasma exchange was first used to treat FH in 1974 at the Hammersmith Hospital, London, [2] and was subsequently adopted in other centres across the world. Initially, fresh-frozen plasma was given as the replacement fluid, but plasma protein fraction (human albumin solution, 4.5%) was used instead from an early stage to minimize allergic reactions in recipients and to maximize reduction of their cholesterol levels. The chief indication for the use of plasma exchange in hypercholesterolaemia is homozygous FH, although plasma exchange has also been used in a small number of heterozygotes and in patients with primary biliary cirrhosis. Three- to 4-litre exchanges carried out in homozygotes weekly or twice monthly over periods of 5–10 years have been shown to improve well-being, induce resolution of xanthomata, and arrest or slow the rate of progression of atheromatous lesions in the root of the aorta and coronary arteries. Regression of atheroma is rare in homozygotes, but was observed in one individual after 5 years of plasma exchange [3].

Comparison of the current ages (or age at death in two instances) of homozygotes treated by plasma exchange with the age at death of their untreated homozygous siblings showed that this procedure significantly prolongs life expectancy, presumably because of the overall halving of LDL cholesterol levels that is achieved, as illustrated in Fig. 13.1. Use of an HMG CoA reductase inhibitor in conjunction with plasma exchange results in an additional 11–12% reduction in pre-exchange cholesterol levels in homozygotes [4].

Plasma exchange is well tolerated and is remarkably free from serious side effects. However, it is unselective in that it not only reduces LDL cholesterol but also other factors that may have a bearing on atherosclerosis including HDL cholesterol. For this reason the idea of selectively removing LDL from plasma has long been an attractive concept, the realization of which in practical terms gave rise to the procedure of LDL apheresis, as discussed below. The non-selectivity of plasma exchange can be advantageous in certain circumstances, however, as when treating primary biliary cirrhosis where the excess cholesterol in plasma is present not as LDL but as Lp-X. The reduction in serum cholesterol achieved by the combined use of plasma exchange

13

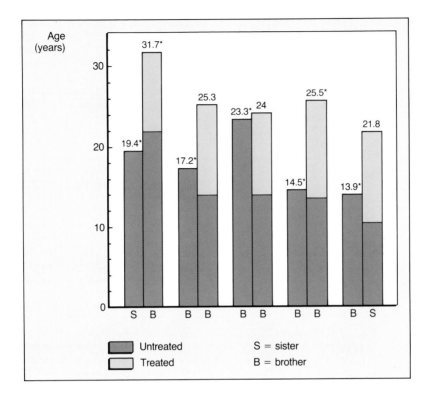

Fig. 13.1. Current ages or *ages at death of five pairs of siblings with homozygous familial hypercholesterolaemia untreated or treated with plasma exchange. Updated from Thompson *et al.*, *Br Med J* 1985, 291:1671–1673.

and lovastatin in such a patient is shown in Fig. 13.2. Another situation where plasma exchange is preferable to LDL apheresis is in the treatment of type V hyperlipoproteinaemia complicated by acute pancreatitis [5]. The rapid reduction of chylomicron and VLDL triglycerides and blood viscosity achieved by this approach is illustrated in Fig. 13.3.

Finally, it is worth pointing out that plasma exchange seems to be just as effective as LDL apheresis in mobilizing tissue cholesterol as judged both by clinical studies of xanthoma regression and experimental studies with radiolabelled cholesterol, despite the acute reduction in HDL cholesterol which occurs after the former procedure. This suggests that reduced influx of LDL cholesterol, which is common to both procedures, is the main determinant of the net decrease in cell cholesterol content rather than changes in HDL-mediated cholesterol efflux.

13

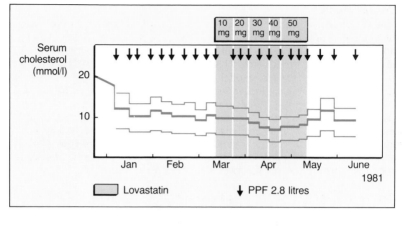

Fig. 13.2. Combined effects of repetitive plasma exchanges with 2.8 l of plasma protein fraction (PPF) and oral lovastatin 10–50 mg/day in a patient with primary biliary cirrhosis. The mean level of serum cholesterol between exchanges is shown by the solid line, together with the immediate pre-exchange (upper line) and post-exchange (lower line) values. Adapted by permission from Thompson, in *Atherosclerosis. Biology and Clinical Science* edited by Olsson AG. Edinburgh: Churchill Livingstone, 1987, pp 431–436.

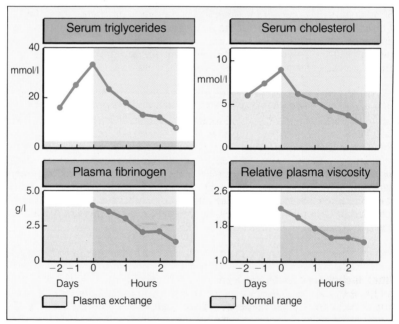

Fig. 13.3. Results of plasma exchange in diabetic with type V hyperlipoproteinaemia and acute pancreatitis. Adapted by permission from Betteridge *et al.*, *Lancet* 1978, i:1368.

13

LDL apheresis

Lupien *et al.* [6] were the first to apply the principle of affinity chromatography to the selective removal of VLDL and LDL. They did this by venesecting FH patients and then mixing batches of their blood with heparin-agarose beads, the blood being reinfused after it had been filtered. This approach was further exploited and refined by Stoffel *et al.* [7], who developed an on-line immunoadsorption column through which plasma from a cell separator could be continuously perfused. Their column consisted of antihuman LDL antibodies raised in sheep and coupled to sepharose. This arrangement proved much more efficient than heparin-agarose beads in reducing LDL cholesterol, mainly because a much larger volume of plasma was treated during each procedure. These columns are not disposable and require sterilization between procedures but can be re-used over long periods of time.

A recent development has been the introduction of disposable chemical affinity columns consisting of dextran sulphate coupled with cellulose [8]. Plasma from which VLDL and LDL is to be removed is separated from blood cells by a hollow-fibre filter and then perfused through the adsorbent column and returned to the patient. As with the immunoadsorbent columns, there is no significant binding of HDL. Each 400 ml column has the capacity to bind 7.5 g of LDL cholesterol; this amount, however, may be insufficient to control effectively the hypercholesterolaemia of some homozygotes. To overcome this limitation, a twin-column automated system has been developed in which 150 ml columns can be re-used several times during a procedure, desorption of bound LDL [9] from one column being synchronized to coincide with the adsorption cycle of the other column. In theory, there are no limits to the amount of LDL that can be adsorbed from plasma when using this system, other than the constraints imposed by the time available.

A pilot study of the combined use of bi-weekly LDL apheresis and lovastatin 40 mg/day in four FH heterozygotes with severe coronary disease has shown that LDL cholesterol can be reduced by almost 50% and the HDL : LDL cholesterol ratio increased more than twofold by this means, as compared with conventional therapy (Fig. 13.4). These changes were accompanied by a lessening in angina and improved exercise tolerance. Computer-assisted analysis of a coronary lesion in one of these patients showed evidence of partial regression after 18 months of LDL apheresis and treatment with an HMG CoA reductase inhibitor, as illustrated in Fig. 13.5. This approach provides a potential means of inducing regression but needs to be assessed further in a randomized trial.

13

Other techniques

Double filtration plasmapheresis, first used to treat homozygous FH in 1982 [10], is as efficient as LDL apheresis in lowering LDL levels but is much less selective. Appreciable decreases in HDL, fibrinogen, and albumin occur with the double filtration procedure, which thus represents a compromise between LDL apheresis and plasma exchange. As with plasma exchange, albumin re-

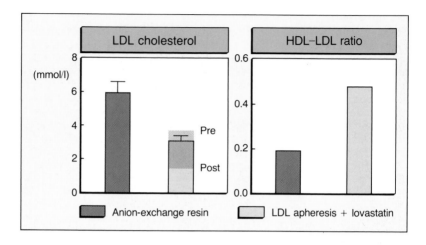

Fig. 13.4. Mean values (± s.e.) of LDL cholesterol and HDL:LDL ratio in four FH heterozygotes on conventional therapy with anion-exchange resin (left) and during bi-weekly LDL apheresis plus lovastatin 20–40 mg/day (right). Changes in LDL cholesterol immediately before (pre) and after (post) LDL apheresis are shown, together with the mean value during the 2 weeks between procedures, obtained by integrating beneath sequential rebound curves.

placements are required, although in smaller quantities. The chief problem with double filtration is the adherence of plasma components to the pores of the second filter, which hinders free passage of HDL and albumin.

The most recent innovation in this field is on-line precipitation of LDL through the addition of heparin to plasma, the so-called Heparin Extracorporeal LDL Precipitation (HELP) system [11]. Precipitation of LDL occurs without addition of cations if the pH is sufficiently low. The precipitate is removed by filtration and the plasma is subsequently dialysed against bicarbonate buffer to restore the pH to normal. LDL is removed efficiently by this process but so is fibrinogen. It remains to be shown whether the latter result has a beneficial effect on atherosclerosis. All forms of extracorporeal cholesterol removal result in marked reductions in Lp(a), greater than can be achieved by other means [12]. It remains to be shown whether it is necessary to reduce both LDL and Lp(a) where raised levels of each co-exist or whether reduction of LDL levels alone is sufficient to render Lp(a) innocuous.

13

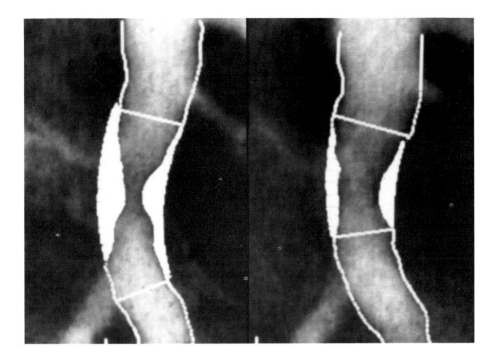

Fig. 13.5. Computer-assisted reconstruction of angiograms showing stenotic lesion in proximal left circumflex artery before (left) and after 18 months of LDL apheresis and lovastatin (right). Adapted by permission from Barbir *et al.*, *Br Med J* 1989, 298:132.

Surgical procedures

Partial ileal bypass

Buchwald [13] was the first to perform partial ileal bypass for hypercholesterolaemia. The procedure involves bypassing the terminal one-third or 200 cm of the ileum, whichever is the greater, by sectioning the ileum and anastomosing its proximal cut-end to the side of the caecum, the distal cut-end being closed. This diverts the intestinal contents away from the sites of absorption of both vitamin B_{12} and bile salts and necessitates lifelong injections of vitamin B_{12}, 1000 µg every 3 months. Postoperative diarrhoea can sometimes be severe but is usually controllable with codeine phosphate or

13

cholestyramine. No other serious side effects have been reported and the procedure seems free from the complications which accompanied the jejunal-ileal bypass operation used to treat obesity. However, mild steatorrhoea, a significant increase in urinary oxalate excretion and a decrease in calcium absorption have all been reported.

The main result of bypassing the ileum is a fourfold increase in bile acid excretion which leads to an increased rate of turnover of cholesterol to bile acids and a compensatory increase in cholesterol synthesis. Studies of LDL turnover in heterozygotes show that LDL catabolism is stimulated more markedly by partial ileal bypass than by cholestyramine, possibly because the former increases bile acid excretion to a greater extent [14]. Interestingly, the increase in LDL catabolism is almost entirely due to an increase in receptor-mediated catabolism [15]. This suggests that increases in bile acid synthesis lead to an increased demand for cholesterol by the liver which is met by an increased rate of LDL uptake via hepatic LDL receptors, as well as by an increase in endogenous cholesterol synthesis.

The chief clinical indication for partial ileal bypass used to be patients with heterozygous FH who were intolerant of anion-exchange resins. However, the advent of HMG CoA reductase inhibitors, either alone or in combination with a small dose of anion-exchange resins, has meant that there are now fewer patients who qualify for the operation on the grounds of drug-resistant hypercholesterolaemia. Nevertheless, there will probably always be some patients who either do not have access to these drugs or in whom side effects preclude their use, and it is therefore worth reviewing briefly past experience with partial ileal bypass. Miettinen and Lempinen [14] showed that it lowered serum cholesterol in heterozygotes to a twofold greater extent than 32 g daily of cholestyramine. Spengel *et al.* [15] studied eight heterozygotes, in whom the serum cholesterol fell by 25% on 16 g daily of cholestyramine and by 38% 2 months after partial ileal bypass. LDL cholesterol initially fell by 36% postoperatively but HDL cholesterol did not change. Subsequent follow-up over a 3-year period showed rises in both LDL and HDL, resulting overall in a favourable increase in the HDL ratio. The rise in LDL cholesterol can be counteracted by concomitant administration of an HMG CoA reductase inhibitor [4].

Information on the effects of partial ileal bypass on coronary atherosclerosis is scanty but two angiographic surveys have been reported. In the first, 22 patients underwent coronary angiography before and $3\frac{1}{2}$ years after partial ileal bypass; lesions progressed in 23%, regressed in 14% and did not change in the remainder. The second series involved patients studied before and 2 years postoperatively, most of whom showed angiographic progression despite a 48% reduction in serum cholesterol. Koivisto and Miettinen [16] recently completed a 10-year follow-up of 27 patients after partial ileal bypass and reported that the incidence of new events and death from CHD did not differ from a group of matched, medically treated patients. Thus, although partial ileal bypass is undoubtedly an effective means of controlling hyper-

13

cholesterolaemia, evidence that this exerts a favourable impact on established CHD is, at best, equivocal.

In contrast to heterozygotes the operation has proved disappointing in controlling the hypercholesterolaemia of FH homozygotes. In some instances serum cholesterol levels actually rose, and it would therefore seem inadvisable to use partial ileal bypass to treat homozygotes.

In a significant percentage of patients the procedure needs to be reversed usually because of persistent diarrhoea or recurrent abdominal pain. Hypercholesterolaemia recrudesces but can usually be brought under control by administration of an HMG CoA reductase inhibitor, as illustrated in Fig. 13.6.

Portacaval shunt

Portacaval shunt was first used to treat an FH homozygote in 1973. This patient responded with a remarkable 60% fall in serum cholesterol and a decrease in the gradient across her aortic valve, but died suddenly 18 months later. Starzl et al. [17] reviewed their experiences with this patient and nine other homozygotes, eight of whom were aged 2–14 years. The average reduction in serum cholesterol was 34% and, although there was little evidence of any serious side effects of the operation itself, three of the patients, all of whom had pre-existing CHD, died within 3 years. Forman et al. [18] followed up 13 homozygotes who had undergone the same procedure up to 6 years previously, and reported a mean decrease in LDL cholesterol of only 18%. None of the patients achieved cholesterol levels of less than 12 mmol/l (460 mg/dl) but xanthomata regressed in eight out of 12. Mild abnormalities of liver function have been observed after portacaval shunting but there has been only one instance of hepatic encephalopathy.

One of the main drawbacks of undertaking this procedure is the variability of response. In several instances, thrombosis of the shunt was held responsible for the failure of the serum cholesterol to fall. The operation is relatively easy to perform, and has the conceptual attraction of counteracting at least one of the metabolic abnormalities responsible for the hypercholesterolaemia of homozygotes, namely the increased synthesis of LDL. However, it has now been outmoded by liver transplantation.

Liver transplantation

The first successful transplantation of the liver from a normal donor into an FH homozygote was reported in 1984 [19]. The patient was a 7-year-old girl with severe CHD who developed episodes of cardiac failure despite previous CABG and who had a heart transplanted at the same time as the liver. Postoperatively her serum cholesterol decreased from a level of over 25 mmol/l to less than 7 mmol/l and this was accompanied by regression of tendon xanthomata. Subsequently, stimulation of the LDL receptors in the

13

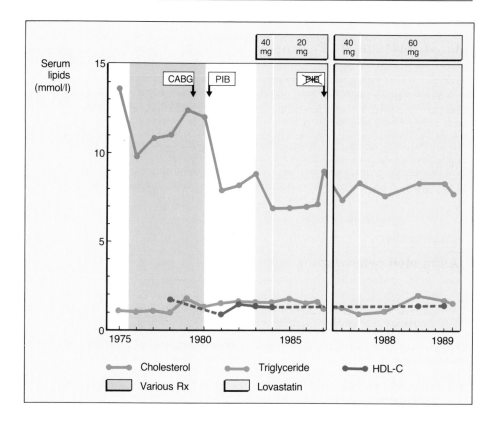

Fig. 13.6. Changes in serum lipids in FH heterozygote after coronary artery bypass grafting (CABG) and following creation of partial ileal bypass (PIB) and its subsequent reversal, and their relation to lovastatin therapy.

donor liver with lovastatin resulted in complete normalization of serum and LDL cholesterol in this patient [20].

Since then at least two other successful liver transplants have been reported. This operation represents the most definitive treatment for homozygous FH currently available. However, it is not without risk, including those risks associated with the long-term use of cyclosporin for immunosuppression.

13

Gene replacement therapy

Gene therapy is still in the experimental stage and has not yet been used to treat hyperlipidaemia in man. However, its potential is obvious in relation to disorders due to absence of receptors, as in FH, and deficiencies of enzymes such as lipoprotein lipase and LCAT or co-factors such as apoC-II. Already it has been shown that injection of complementary DNA encoding the human LDL receptor into fertilized mouse eggs results in a strain of mice expressing high levels of LDL receptors in their liver [21]. There are still major scientific and ethical problems to be overcome before gene therapy becomes feasible in humans but when the day does arrive the inherited hyperlipidaemias will be high up on the list of candidate diseases.

Annotated references

1.   TURNBERG LA, MAHONEY MP, GLEESON MH, FREEMAN CB, GOWENLOCK AH: **Plasmapheresis and plasma exchange in the treatment of hyperlipidaemia and xanthomatous neuropathy in patients with primary biliary cirrhosis.** *Gut* 1972, 13:976–981.
First description of the use of a cell-separator to undertake plasma exchange for hypercholesterolaemia.

2.   THOMPSON GR, LOWENTHAL R, MYANT NB: **Plasma exchange in the management of homozygous familial hypercholesterolaemia.** *Lancet* 1975, i:1208–1211.
First description of use of plasma exchange to treat homozygous familial hypercholesterolaemia.

3.   THOMPSON GR, BARBIR M, OKABAYASHI K, TRAYNER I, LARKIN S: **Plasmapheresis in familial hypercholesterolemia.** *Arteriosclerosis* 1989, 9 (suppl I):I152–I157.
Review of the pros and cons of plasma exchange and LDL apheresis in the management of familial hypercholesterolaemia.

4.   THOMPSON GR, FORD J, JENKINSON M, TRAYNER I: **Efficacy of mevinolin as adjuvant therapy for refractory familial hypercholesterolaemia.** *Q J Med* 1986, 60:803–811.
Initial experience with lovastatin (mevinolin) in the management of severe familial hypercholesterolaemia.

5.   RICHTER WO, BREHM G, SCHWANDT P: **Type V hyperlipoproteinemia and plasmapheresis.** *Ann Intern Med* 1987, 106:779.
Description of two patients with acute pancreatitis complicating severe hypertriglyceridaemia who were successfully treated with plasma exchange.

6.   LUPIEN P-J, MOORJANI S, AWAD J: **A new approach to the management of familial hypercholesterolaemia: removal of plasma cholesterol based on the principle of affinity chromatography.** *Lancet* 1976, i:1261–1265.
First use of heparin-agarose beads to adsorb LDL selectively from whole blood.

13

7.   STOFFEL W, BORBERG H, GREVE V: Application of specific extracorporeal removal of low density lipoprotein in familial hypercholesterolaemia. *Lancet* 1981, ii:1005–1007.
First description of LDL apheresis in man using immunoadsorption columns.

8.   YOKOYAMA S, HAYASHI R, SATANI M, YAMAMOTO A: Selective removal of low density lipoprotein by plasmapheresis in familial hypercholesterolemia. *Arteriosclerosis* 1985, 5:613–622.
First description of use of disposable dextran sulphate-cellulose columns to undertake LDL apheresis.

9.   MABUCHI H, MICHISHITA I, TAKEDA M, FUJITA H, KOIZUMI J, TAKEDA R, TAKADA S, OONISHI M: A new low density lipoprotein apheresis system using two dextran sulfate cellulose columns in an automated column regenerating unit (LDL continuous apheresis). *Atherosclerosis* 1987, 68:19–26.
Modification of system described in [8].

10.   HOMMA Y, MIKAMI Y, TAMACHI H, NAKAYA N, NAKAMURA H, GOTO Y: Comparison of selectivity of LDL removal by double filtration and dextran-sulfate cellulose column plasmapheresis, and changes of subfractionated plasma lipoproteins after plasmapheresis in heterozygous familial hypercholesterolemia. *Metabolism* 1987, 36:419–425.
Comparison of double filtration and dextran sulphate column methods of performing LDL apheresis.

11.   FUCHS C, WINDISCH M, WIELAND H, ARMSTRONG VW, RIEGER J, KOSTERING H, SCHELER F, SEIDEL D: Selective continuous extracorporeal elimination of low density lipoproteins from plasma by heparin precipitation without cations. In *Plasma Separation and Plasma Fractionation*. Basel: Karger, 1983, pp 272–280.
Description of the HELP system of LDL apheresis.

12.   SCHENCK I, KELLER CH, HAILER S, WOLFRAM G, ZÖLLNER N: Reduction of Lp(a) by different methods of plasma exchange. *Klin Wochenschr* 1988, 66:1197–1201.
Studies in FH patients which suggest that plasma exchange or HELP apheresis reduce Lp(a) levels to a similar extent, although only half as efficiently as they reduce LDL levels.

13.   BUCHWALD H: Lowering of cholesterol absorption and blood levels by ileal exclusion. *Circulation* 1964, 29:713–720.
Mentions first instance of partial ileal bypass undertaken in a human to treat hypercholesterolaemia.

14.   MIETTINEN TA, LEMPINEN M: Cholestyramine and ileal bypass in the treatment of familial hypercholesterolaemia. *Eur J Clin Invest* 1977, 7:509–514.
Comparison of effects of cholestyramine and partial ileal bypass on serum cholesterol and faecal steroids in FH.

15.   SPENGEL FA, JADHAV A, DUFFIELD RGM, WOOD CB, THOMPSON GR: Cholesterol reduction in familial hypercholesterolaemia: superiority of partial ileal bypass over cholestyramine. *Lancet* 1981, ii:768–770.
Comparison of effects of cholestyramine and partial ileal bypass on turnover of native and cyclohexanedione-linked LDL in FH heterozygotes.

13

16.   KOIVISTO P, MIETTINEN TA: **Long-term effects of ileal bypass on lipoproteins in patients with familial hypercholesterolemia.** *Circulation* 1984, 70:290–296.
Assessment of the rather disappointing results of partial ileal bypass in 27 FH heterozygotes followed up for 10 years.

17.   STARZL TE, CHASE HP, AHRENS EH, MCNAMARA DJ, BILHEIMER DW, SCHAEFER EJ, REY J, PORTER KA, STEIN E, FRANCAVILLA A, BENSON LN: **Portacaval shunt in patients with familial hypercholesterolaemia.** *Ann Surg* 1983, 198:273–283.
Review of results of portacaval shunt in 10 FH homozygotes.

18.   FORMAN MB, BAKER SG, MIENY CJ, JOFFE BI, SANDLER MP, MENDELSOHN D, SEFTEL HC: **Treatment of homozygous familial hypercholesterolaemia with portacaval shunt.** *Atherosclerosis* 1982, 41:349–361.
Results of portacaval shunts for homozygous FH carried out in South Africa.

19.   STARZL TE, BILHEIMER DW, BAHNSON HT, SHAW BW, HARDESTY RL, GRIFFITH BP, IWATSUKI S, ZITELLI BJ, GARTNER JC, MALATACK JJ, URBACH AH: **eart-liver transplantation in a patient with familial hypercholesterolaemia.** *Lancet* 1984, i:1382–1383.
Description of a remarkable 'first': combined heart-liver transplantation in an FH homozygote.

20.   EAST C, GRUNDY SM, BILHEIMER DW: **Normal cholesterol levels with lovastatin (mevinolin) therapy in a child with homozygous familial hypercholesterolemia following liver transplantation.** *JAMA* 1986, 256:2843–2848.
Response to lovastatin of patient described in [19].

21.   HOFMANN SL, RUSSELL DW, BROWN MS, GOLDSTEIN JL, HAMMER RE: **Overexpression of low density lipoprotein (LDL) receptor eliminates LDL from plasma in transgenic mice.** *Science* 1988, 239:1277–1281.
Successful introduction of functioning human LDL receptors into transgenic mice.

13

14 DETECTION OF HYPERLIPIDAEMIA AND BENEFITS OF TREATMENT

Frequency of hyperlipidaemia and coronary heart disease

Screening for hyperlipidaemia

Policy statements on intervention

Practical guidelines for the clinician

Evidence that treatment of hyperlipidaemia influences coronary heart disease

Proposals for the future
Professional training in lipidology
Creation of more lipid clinics
Increasing the level of awareness

Annotated references

Frequency of hyperlipidaemia and coronary heart disease

As discussed in Chapter 5 the incidence of CHD varies widely between different countries, as does the prevalence of hypercholesterolaemia with which it is so closely correlated. Here we will focus on the frequency of this disease and its harbinger in the British population, which is near the top of the world ratings in both respects.

The major causes of death in England and Wales during 1987 are shown in Fig. 14.1. CHD was responsible in 31% of males and 24% of females, a total of over 150 000 deaths per year. Unlike the USA there has been only a very small decline in mortality from CHD during the past 20 years in Britain. One possible explanation for this discrepancy is that although decreases in smoking have occurred to a similar extent in both countries, changes in diet have been far more marked and widespread in the USA [1]. It is significant that hypercholesterolaemia is now more than twice as common in middle-aged men in Britain as in North America [2].

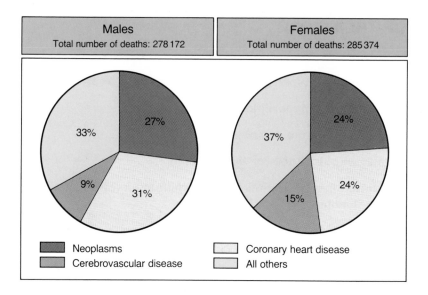

Fig. 14.1. Proportion of all deaths in England and Wales (1987) attributed to coronary heart disease, cerebrovascular disease, neoplasms and all other causes. Source: Office of Population Censuses and Surveys.

The prevalence of CHD in Britain, estimated on the basis of symptoms or electrocardiographic evidence of myocardial ischaemia, appears to be around 20% in men aged 50–60, judging from the Whitehall Study [3] and the more recent British Regional Heart Study [4]. Half the deaths observed in prospective studies occur in such individuals. The mortality from CHD in men of this age is around 1% per annum so that if premature death is defined as dying before 65 then approximately 15% of men over the age of 50 will die prematurely from CHD. The age-adjusted rate in females is about one-third that of males.

A high proportion of individuals dying from CHD would have been hypercholesterolaemic during life and therefore identifiable as being at increased risk. However, as illustrated in Table 14.1, 75% of these deaths occur in the 50% of the population which has a serum cholesterol in the range 5.7–8.0 mmol/l, whereas only 15% occur in the 5% of the population with a serum cholesterol > 8.0 mmol/l, notwithstanding the much greater relative risk within the latter category. The fact that only 10% of CHD deaths occur in the 45% of the population with a cholesterol < 5.7 mmol/l speaks for itself. Although these data relate to men studied in Framingham during the 1960s they are probably applicable to contemporary Britain in that the distribution of cholesterol in Britons now is similar to that of Americans then.

14

Table 14.1. Relationship between serum cholesterol and CHD mortality.

Serum cholesterol (mmol/l)	Population (%)	Attributable CHD deaths (%)
<5.7	45	10
5.7–8.0	50	75
>8.0	5	15

Data from Blackburn *et al.*, *Circulation* 1987, (suppl 1):165–167.

The frequency distribution of serum cholesterol in British men and women undergoing health screening is shown in Fig. 14.2. Although this sample of the population is largely self-selected, the bias that this introduces appears to be small in that the mean serum cholesterol of men aged 40–59 screened in 1984 was identical to that of men of the same age surveyed during the British Regional Heart Study (6.3 mmol/l), which was more representative of the population as a whole. Data from another survey are given in Table 14.2, which shows that a significant degree of hypercholesterolaemia (>6.5 mmol/l) is present in a quarter of adult men and women below the age of 60. In contrast, hypertension was present in 10–15% and hyperglycaemia in only 1%.

Table 14.2. Prevalence of risk factors for CHD in 12 092 Britons aged 25–59.

Risk factor	Men	Women
Cholesterol		
>8.0 mmol/l	4%	4%
>6.5 mmol/l	26%	24%
Family history of CHD	36%	40%
Smoking	38%	31%
Blood pressure > 160/90 mmHg	15%	10%
Fasting glucose >7 mmol/l	1%	1%

Data calculated from [8].

Screening for hyperlipidaemia

The magnitude of the problems caused by CHD and the frequency of hypercholesterolaemia raise the obvious question of whether widespread screening for this risk factor should be undertaken in an effort to prevent premature disability and death from that disorder.

14

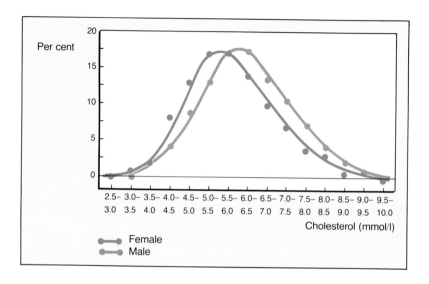

Fig. 14.2. Frequency distribution of serum cholesterol in men (n = 8272) and women (n = 8136) aged 20–70 screened at the British United Provident Association (BUPA) Medical Centre, London, during 1987. The mean (s.d.) was 6.2 (1.2) mmol/l in men and 5.8 (1.2) mmol/l in women, over 80% of both sexes being aged 30–59. The 75th, 90th and 95th percentile values for each sex were 6.9 and 6.5, 7.7 and 7.4, and 8.2 and 7.9 mmol/l, respectively. The percentages of men and women with values between 5.2 and 6.5, 6.5 and 7.8, and >7.8 mmol/l were 43 and 41%, 26 and 18%, and 9 and 6%, respectively. Published by permission of Dr C. Ritchie.

The advantages and pitfalls of mass screening have recently been summarized in a statement from the US National Cholesterol Education Program [5]. This points out the necessity of a simple yet accurate and reliable means of measurement, to avoid the problems arising from falsely low or high values; the logistical difficulty of coping with large numbers of individuals at one time; and the need to provide nutritional guidance on-site and access to specialist advice. Add to this the considerable cost involved and it is clear that screening the entire population, although possibly desirable, is an endeavour not to be entered into lightly.

Alternative approaches to screening have also been advocated. The first involves opportunistic screening of all individuals who attend their general practitioner for whatever reason, preferably on the first occasion that the patient is seen as an adult [6]. This approach is analogous to that taken by many general practitioners in detecting hypertension. The second approach is to screen selectively all those regarded as being at high risk on account of

14

a family history of premature CHD or the presence of hypercholesterolaemia in a first-degree relative [1,7].

At the very least it is advocated that screening should be undertaken in all individuals in whom the likelihood of hyperlipidaemia is high, or in whom other risk factors are present (Table 14.3). This should enable the majority of individuals with a serum cholesterol >8 mmol/l to be identified although none of the criteria listed has a high specificity on its own [8]. The development of easier ways of measuring serum lipids (see Chapter 3) and the increasing interest in prevention among the public as well as the medical profession should help facilitate the detection of hyperlipidaemia. Eventually it may be possible to achieve what is arguably the ideal state of affairs where every adult will have had their serum lipids measured at least once before they reach the age of 30. Current estimates are that less than 10% of the British population has ever had their cholesterol measured.

Table 14.3 Selective screening for hyperlipidaemia.

1	First-degree relatives of known hyperlipidaemics
2	Xanthelasma or xanthomata
3	Corneal arcus before 60
4	Family history of CHD before 60
5	Hypertension
6	Diabetes
7	Chronic renal disease
8	Known CHD, PVD or CVD, including post-CABG and angioplasty

PVD, peripheral vascular disease; CVD, cerebrovascular disease.

Policy statements on intervention

At least five separate policy statements have been published during the past 5 years aimed at establishing practical guidelines for defining hypercholesterolaemia in relation to risk of CHD and suggesting appropriate methods of intervention. Because the criteria have changed during that period it is logical to consider these statements in chronological order.

1985. The NIH Consensus Development Conference Statement [6] stratified cholesterol into moderate-risk and high-risk categories according to age-related 75th and 90th percentiles for the US population. The cut-offs used were values above 5.2, 5.7 and 6.2 for moderate risk in those aged 20–29, 30–39 and 40 years and above, respectively, the corresponding high-risk values being 5.7, 6.2 and 6.7 mmol/l. Dietary therapy was recommended for both grades of hypercholesterolaemia with the option of adding drugs in those in

14

the high-risk category. No recommendations were made about hypertriglyceridaemia.

1987. The British Cardiac Society (BCS) advocated giving dietary advice to individuals with a serum cholesterol above 6.5 mmol/l, supplemented, if necessary, with drugs in those with a value above 7.8 mmol/l, with the aim of lowering the level to 5.2 mmol/l [1].

The European Atherosclerosis Society (EAS) recommended dietary advice in those with a serum cholesterol between 5.2–6.5 mmol/l, with the option of adding drug therapy in those with a cholesterol > 6.5 mmol/l or a cholesterol > 5.2 mmol/l and a triglyceride > 2.3 mmol/l [9]. The EAS recommendations took account of other risk factors in assessing risk, including a family history of CHD, male sex, youthful age, a low HDL cholesterol (< 0.9 mmol/l), and classic risk factors such as diabetes, hypertension and smoking.

The British Hyperlipidaemia Association (BHA) guidelines were a compromise between those of the BCS and the EAS but pointed out that hypercholesterolaemia due solely to hyperαlipoproteinaemia (HDL cholesterol > 2 mmol/l) did not require treatment and stressed the need for vigorous treatment of hyperlipidaemia in patients with established CHD, especially those who had undergone coronary artery bypass grafting or angioplasty [10]. Another recommendation was that persistent hypertriglyceridaemia (> 3 mmol/l) in the presence of a low HDL cholesterol (< 1 mmol/l) required treatment.

1988. The most recent policy statement is that by the Expert Panel of the US National Cholesterol Education Program (NCEP) which proposed a classification of hypercholesterolaemia based on total and LDL cholesterol values, unrelated to age. Total cholesterol was defined as 'desirable' (< 5.2 mmol/l), 'borderline–high' (5.2–6.2 mmol/l) and 'high' (> 6.2 mmol/l). Calculation of LDL cholesterol, based on measurement of total and HDL cholesterol and triglyceride, was advocated in all those with a 'high' total cholesterol and those in the 'borderline–high' category who had either CHD or two additional risk factors. The latter included all those mentioned in the EAS report plus severe obesity (> 30% overweight) and a history of cerebrovascular or peripheral vascular disease [11].

The NCEP report included detailed recommendations on dietary therapy (see Chapter 11) and the use of LDL cholesterol as a guide to drug therapy. The latter was advised in those who, despite diet, had an LDL cholesterol > 4.9 mmol/l or who had a value of 4.1 mmol/l together with CHD or two other risk factors.

14

Practical guidelines for the clinician

In an attempt to achieve a simplified consensus of all these statements the following approach to the detection and management of hyperlipidaemia is proposed, always bearing in mind that young, male patients offer the greatest scope for intervention and that the risks of long-term drug therapy are easier to justify in patients with established CHD than in asymptomatic patients.

A suggested scheme of investigation is set out in Table 14.4 and the interpretation of results obtained is shown in Table 14.5. For the sake of simplicity, the latter ignores the effects of age and sex, even though these can be considerable (see Chapter 1).

Table 14.4. Scheme of investigation.

1	Do random total cholesterol
2	If values <5.2 mmol/l, reassure and repeat in 5 years
(a)	If value 5.2–6.5 mmol/l, give general dietary advice
(b)	If value 5.2–6.5 mmol/l and patient has CHD or 2 other risk factors, or if value >6.5 mmol/l:

—   measure fasting total cholesterol, triglyceride, HDL cholesterol

—   calculate LDL cholesterol as:
LDLC = TC − HDLC − (TG / 2.2) mmol/l
(unless TG > 4.5)

—   calculate HDL ratio as:
HDL ratio = HDLC / (TC − HDLC)

Table 14.5. Interpretation of results.

mmol/l serum	Desirable	Borderline	Abnormal
Total cholesterol	<5.2	5.2–6.5	>6.5
LDL cholesterol	<4.0	4.0–5.0	>5.0
HDL cholesterol	>1.0	0.9–1.0	<0.9
Triglyceride	<2.0	2.0–2.5	>2.5
HDL ratio	>0.25	0.2–0.25	<0.2

A rapid scheme for determining lipoprotein phenotype is shown in Table 14.6. Methods of discriminating between types III, IV and V are given in Chapter 4.

Proposals for assessing the degree of risk and the appropriate therapeutic response are shown in Tables 14.7 and 14.8.

14

Table 14.6. Lipoprotein phenotypes.

TC	LDLC	HDLC	TG	Phenotype
↑	↑	↑, ↓or N	N	IIa
↑	↑	↑, ↓or N	↑	IIb
↑or N	N or ↓	↑, ↓or N	↑	III, IV or V
↑	N	↑	N	Hyperαlipoproteinaemia

Table 14.7. Assessment of risk.

1   Lipid risk factors are: Abnormal (high) total or LDL cholesterol
                                Abnormal (high) total triglyceride and/or
                                Abnormal (low) HDL cholesterol
    Other risk factors are: Male sex
                                Family history of CHD before 60
                                Hypertension
                                Smoking
                                Hyperglycaemia

2   *Moderate risk* is defined as one lipid risk factor plus not more than
    one other risk factor

    High risk is defined as two lipid risk factors (total cholesterol
    >7.8 mmol/l counts as two), or one lipid risk factor and two other
    risk factors, or one lipid risk factor and CHD. Reversibility of risk is
    greater if age < 40.

3   Alternatively, calculate arbitrary risk factor score based on severity
    of hypercholesterolaemia and other risk factors [12] or calculate
    Framingham multifactorial logistic function (see ref. [19] in chapter 5)

Evidence that treatment of hyperlipidaemia influences CHD

There are three lines of evidence which have a bearing on this question:
international or regional changes in CHD mortality in relation to changes
in risk factors over time; effects of treating hyperlipidaemia on the clinical
manifestations of CHD in prevention trials; and the impact of lipid-lowering
measures on the rate of progression of coronary atherosclerosis, gauged angiographically. The latter topic was dealt with in Chapter 6 and will not be
considered further except to reiterate that the results of recent angiographic
trials support the notion that lipid-lowering therapy is beneficial.

14

Table 14.8. Therapeutic recommendations.

1   Institute dietary therapy via dietician in all instances except
    hyperalipoproteinaemia, where reassurance is all that is required

2   Use drugs only in high-risk patients in whom diet fails to bring lipids
    out of abnormal range

3   Suggested drug regimens:
    Type IIa   Anion exchange resin, fibrate or HMG CoA reductase inhibitor
    Type IIb   Anion exchange resin plus fibrate or nicotinic acid, or
                HMG CoA reductase inhibitor ± fibrate with caution
    Type III   Fibrate or HMG CoA reductase inhibitor
    Type IV   Fibrate or nicotinic acid
    Type V   Nicotinic acid, Maxepa or fibrate

Changing trends in coronary heart disease in certain countries also support the idea that a reduction in serum cholesterol is worthwhile. For example, there has been a 30% decrease in CHD mortality in the USA since 1968. One reason for this is the 0.6–0.8 mmol/l decrease in serum cholesterol which occurred between 1960 and 1980, possibly reflecting changing dietary habits [13]. The decreased mortality reflects a reduced incidence of the disease, not just a decrease in the case fatality rate. As a result the USA now has only the tenth highest CHD mortality rate in the world, having been second only to Finland in 1967.

Since 1978 the results of six major trials of lipid-lowering therapy in the prevention of CHD which have given a positive result have been published. Four of these have been trials of primary prevention [14–17], two have involved secondary intervention [18,19]. All except one of these trials has been reviewed in detail elsewhere [20,21] the exception being the Stockholm Secondary Prevention Trial, which has only recently been published [19]. This was a non-blind trial involving 555 survivors of a myocardial infarct less than 70 years old. All were given dietary and anti-smoking advice and were then randomized into a control and a treatment group, the latter receiving clofibrate 2 g and nicotinic acid 3 g daily for 5 years. During this period values of serum cholesterol and triglyceride were 13 and 19% lower, respectively, in the treatment group than in the controls. These changes were associated with a 36% reduction in CHD mortality ($P < 0.01$) and a 26% reduction in total mortality ($P < 0.05$). The results of all six trials are summarized in Table 14.9.

Significant decreases in CHD occurred in all of them but decreases in total mortality were observed only in the two secondary prevention trials. In the Coronary Drug Project this did not become significant until nine years after the end of the trial. In the WHO trial of clofibrate total mortality increased during and after the trial, whereas in the other three primary prevention trials it did not change. In the Stockholm trial the reduction in CHD was attributed

14

Table 14.9. Major lipid-lowering trials of CHD prevention, 1978–1988.

Trial	Treatment	Duration (years)	TC	TG	HDL-C	Outcome
Primary						
Oslo	Diet and anti-smoking	5	−20%	−29%	—	45% ↓all CHD
WHO	Clofibrate	5.3	−9%	—	—	25% ↓non-fatal CHD 25% ↑total mortality*
LRC-CPPT	Cholestyramine	7	−12%	+17%	+6%	19% ↓all CHD
Helsinki Heart Study	Gemfibrozil	5	−9%	−35%	+9%	34% ↓all CHD
Secondary						
Coronary Drug Project	Nicotinic acid	6.2	−9%	−27%	—	12% ↓fatal CHD[†] 11% ↓total mortality[†]
Stockholm Trial	Clofibrate + nicotinic acid	5	−13%	−19%	—	36% ↓fatal CHD 26% ↓total mortality
Mean change			−12%	−19%	+7.5%	29% ↓CHD

*After 9.6 years; [†]after 15 years.

to the decrease in triglyceride not cholesterol, but changes in HDL cholesterol were not examined. Even greater reductions in serum triglyceride were observed in the Helsinki Heart Study but the reduction in CHD was ascribed entirely to the accompanying decreases in LDL cholesterol and increases in HDL cholesterol. In the LRC trial triglycerides rose and the reduction in CHD was attributed mainly to decreases in LDL cholesterol.

Overall the average reduction in CHD in these six trials was 29%, which was associated with mean decreases in total cholesterol and triglyceride of 12 and 19%, respectively; in two trials these changes were accompanied by a mean increase in HDL cholesterol of 7.5%. The corresponding changes in the concentration of each of these lipids were −0.8, −0.4 and +0.09 mmol/l. Thus, relatively small changes in serum lipids achieved by diet or drugs can reduce the combined morbidity and mortality from CHD by almost one-third over a period of 5–6 years; this is accompanied by a reduction in total mortality in those with pre-existing CHD. Statistical analysis by Peto of the results of these and various other diet and drug trials indicates that for every 1% decrease in serum cholesterol there is a 2% reduction in CHD risk [22]. It remains to be confirmed, however, whether reductions in triglyceride and increases in HDL cholesterol bring additional benefit.

14

Proposals for the future

Professional training in lipidology

There is a lamentable lack of knowledge of lipidology among members of the public or the medical profession in most countries, mainly due to inadequate training. This could be remedied if a short spell of postgraduate education and practical instruction in lipidology were included in the training requirements of all physicians specializing in cardiology, endocrinology, clinical pharmacology and metabolic medicine. Others who might benefit are clinical biochemists and community physicians. Inclusion of the topic in the undergraduate curriculum and in refresher courses should eventually result in better informed general practitioners, which is vital if hyperlipidaemia is to be detected before it does its damage.

Creation of more lipid clinics

As larger numbers of subjects are screened, so there will be an increased demand for referral of severe or refractory cases of hyperlipidaemia for specialist advice. In Britain the few lipid clinics that exist do so on an *ad hoc* basis, with little or no permanent financial support, and no career structure for those who staff them, yet despite these handicaps they fulfil an important role. Every large hospital with a cardiac unit should have one, especially if it undertakes cardiac surgery. Creation of more lipid clinics could be an important step towards reducing the burden of CHD in the community.

Increasing the level of awareness

An attempt was made five years ago by the Committee on the Medical Aspects of Food Policy (COMA) to alert the British to the dangers of hyperlipidaemia and the need to eat a better diet [7] but this advice appears to have gone largely unheeded. The apathy may have been due to the message being delivered in too low a key to reach members of the public and the evidence behind it may not have been persuasive enough for their doctors. However, the recent evidence of benefit from intervention makes it increasingly difficult to sustain the attitude of masterly inactivity which is exemplified in the following extract from a letter of referral, sent by an enlightened general practitioner.

'Mr S. is a 38-year-old man who underwent an extensive coronary artery bypass operation in December 1987. His postoperative recovery was physically uneventful; however, we were quite concerned about our inability to reduce his high cholesterol and triglyceride levels. Up until August 1988 he was taking Questran six a day and Maxepa 5 ml twice daily. On that regime his cholesterols were 8.4–9.5 mmol/l, triglycerides 3.3–5.3 mmol/l.

'Mr S. was getting very screwed up about his inability to drop his cholesterol and triglycerides and was very frightened that his new coronary ar-

14

teries (*sic*) were soon to get furred up. As a result of this I referred him to the...Hospital. He saw a consultant at that hospital who told him to forget taking any tablets, to forget his cholesterol and triglycerides and to go away and try and live a normal life. That advice caused us some considerable concern, especially as we have been working very hard on him over the last couple of years to reduce these levels. He is now on no medication.'

Hopefully, the therapeutic nihilism towards hyperlipidaemia advocated by the consultant in that letter (who worked in a noted cardiothoracic centre) will soon become a thing of the past. Certainly there is greater awareness now of the role of cholesterol in heart disease among both physicians and members of the public in the USA [23,24]. Much of the credit for this must go to those who initiated and maintained the Framingham Study [25], to the National, Heart, Lung, and Blood Institute and the American Heart Association for their leadership and financial support for work in this field and, crucially, to the high quality of research undertaken in academic institutions, which earned Michael Brown and Joseph Goldstein (Department of Molecular Genetics, University of Texas Health Science Center) the 1985 Nobel Prize in Physiology or Medicine.

Annotated references

1.   THE BRITISH CARDIAC SOCIETY WORKING GROUP ON CORONARY PREVENTION: **Conclusions and recommendations**. *Br Heart J* 1987, **57**:188–189.
Summary of the British Cardiac Society's report, which advocates a conservative approach to the management of hypercholesterolaemia.

2.   THOMPSON GR, ROBINSON D, ALLAWAY SL, BEVAN EA, RITCHIE CD: **Prevalence of hyperlipidaemia in British compared with North American men**. In *Expanding Horizons in Atherosclerosis Research* edited by Schlierf G, Mörl H. Berlin: Springer-Verlag, 1987, pp 114–121.
Comparison of serum lipids in men screened by BUPA with plasma lipid values from the LRC Study, duly corrected for methodological differences.

3.   ROSE G, REID DD, HAMILTON PJS, MCCARTNEY P, KEEN H, JARRETT RJ: **Myocardial ischaemia, risk factors and death from coronary heart disease**. *Lancet* 1977, **i**:105–109.
Five-year follow up of over 18 000 civil servants which analyses CHD mortality in relation to risk factors.

4.   SHAPER AG, POCOCK SJ, WALKER M, PHILLIPS AN, WHITEHEAD TP, MACFARLANE PW: **Risk factors for ischaemic heart disease: the prospective phase of the British Regional Heart Study**. *J Epidemiol Community Health* 1985, **39**:197–209.
Epidemiological data on almost 8000 men which examines regional variations in CHD in relation to risk factors.

14

5.   NATIONAL CHOLESTEROL EDUCATION PROGRAM: **Public screening strategies for mea-suring blood cholesterol in adults — issues for special concern.** US Department of Health and Human Services, National Institutes of Health: Office of of Prevention, Education, and Control, National Heart, Lung, and Blood Institute, 1988.
An appraisal of the pros and cons of mass screening.

6.   CONSENSUS CONFERENCE: **Lowering blood cholesterol to prevent heart disease.** *JAMA* 1985, **253**:2080–2086.
The now-superseded statement by the NIH Consensus Development Conference.

7.   COMMITTEE ON MEDICAL ASPECTS OF FOOD POLICY: **Diet and cardiovascular disease.** Department of Health and Social Security, Report on Health and Social Services 28. London: HM Stationery Office, 1984.
Statement from the COMA panel on diet in relation to cardiovascular disease in Britain.

8.   MANN JI, LEWIS B, SHEPHERD J, WINDER AF, FENSTER S, ROSE L, MORGAN B: **Blood lipid concentrations and other cardiovascular risk factors: distribution, preva-lence and detection in Britain.** *Br Med J* 1988, **296**:1702–1706.
Data on risk factors for cardiovascular disease in subjects recruited from general practition-ers' lists in Glasgow, Leicester, London and Oxford.

9.   STUDY GROUP, EUROPEAN ATHEROSCLEROSIS SOCIETY: **Strategies for the prevention of coronary heart disease: a policy statement of the European Atherosclerosis Society.** *Eur Heart J* 1987, **8**:77–88.
A detailed statement on the detection and management of CHD compiled and promulgated under the aegis of the EAS.

10.   SHEPHERD J, BETTERIDGE DJ, DURRINGTON P, LAKER M, LEWIS B, MANN J, MILLER JP, RECKLESS JPD, THOMPSON GR: **Strategies for reducing coronary heart disease and desirable limits for blood lipid concentrations: guidelines of the British Hyper-lipidaemia Association.** *Br Med J* 1987, **295**:1245–1246.
Brief set of proposals aimed at clarifying the definition and indications for treatment of hyperlipidaemia in Britain.

11.   NATIONAL CHOLESTEROL EDUCATION PROGRAM. **Report of the Expert Panel on detec-tion, evaluation, and treatment of high blood cholesterol in adults.** *Arch Intern Med* 1988, **148**:36–69.
Very detailed proposals on the detection and management of hyperlipidaemia in the USA at present.

12.   ANGGARD EE, LAND JM, LENIHAN CJ, PACKARD CJ, PERCY MJ, RITCHIE LD, SHEPHERD J: **Prevention of cardiovascular disease in general practice: a proposed model.** *Br Med J* 1986, **293**:177–180.
Description of a computerized screening model to aid in the detection and evaluation of risk factors for CHD in general practice.

13.   NATIONAL CENTER FOR HEALTH STATISTICS — NATIONAL HEART, LUNG, AND BLOOD INSTITUTE COLLABORATIVE LIPID GROUP: **Trends in serum cholesterol levels among US adults aged 20 to 74 years.** *JAMA* 1987, **257**:937–942.
Analysis of changes in serum cholesterol within the USA based on surveys carried out over 20 years.

14

14.   REPORT FROM THE COMMITTEE OF PRINCIPAL INVESTIGATORS: **A cooperative trial in the primary prevention of ischaemic heart disease using clofibrate.** *Br Heart J* 1978, **40**:1069–1118.
First report of the results of the WHO trial of clofibrate which showed that the drug prevented non-fatal CHD but caused gallstones.

15.   HJERMANN I, HOLME I, VELVE BYRE K, LEREN P: **Effect of diet and smoking intervention on the incidence of coronary heart disease. Report from the Oslo Study Group of a randomized trial in healthy men.** *Lancet* 1981, **ii**:1303–1310.
Trial which showed that anti-smoking advice and dietary treatment of hypercholesterolaemic men resulted in a significant reduction in the incidence of CHD.

16.   LIPID RESEARCH CLINICS PROGRAM: **The Lipid Research Clinics Coronary Primary Prevention Trial results. 1. Reduction in incidence of coronary heart disease.** *JAMA* 1984, **251**:351–364.
The famous multi-million dollar trial which showed that reduction of LDL cholesterol by cholestyramine significantly decreased morbidity and mortality from CHD.

17.   FRICK MH, ELO O, HAAPA K, HEINONEN OP, HEINSALMI P, HELO P, HUTTUNEN JK, KAITANIEMI P, KOSKINEN P, MANNINEN V, MAENPAA H, MALKONEN M, MANTAARI M, NOROLA S, PASTERNACK A, PIKKARAINEN J, ROMO M, SJOBLOM T, NIKKILA EA: **Helsinki Heart Study: primary prevention trial with gemfibrozil in middle-aged men with dyslipidaemia.** *N Engl J Med* 1987, **317**:1237–1245.
First trial claiming to show that a therapeutically induced increase in HDL cholesterol can help prevent CHD.

18.   CANNER PL, BERGE KG, WENGER NK, STAMLER J, FRIEDMAN L, PRINEAS RJ, FRIEDEWALD W: **Fifteen year mortality in coronary drug project patients: long-term benefit with niacin.** *J Am Coll Cardiol* 1986, **8**:1245–1255.
Long-term follow up of the previously negative results of the Coronary Drug Project which showed that the nicotinic acid group eventually had less CHD and lower total mortality than the placebo group.

19.   CARLSON LA, ROSENHAMER G: **Reduction of mortality in the Stockholm Ischaemic Heart Disease Secondary Prevention Study by combined treatment with clofibrate and nicotinic acid.** *Acta Med Scand* 1988, **223**:405–418.
Secondary prevention drug trial which attributed decreased mortality from CHD and all causes to reduction of triglycerides not cholesterol.

20.   THOMPSON GR: **Evidence that lowering serum lipids favourably influences coronary heart disease.** *Q J Med* 1987, **62**:87–95.
Review of the results of prevention trials and other sources of data showing that lipid-lowering initiatives are worthwhile.

21.   BILHEIMER DW: **Therapeutic control of hyperlipidaemia in the prevention of coronary atherosclerosis: a review of results from recent clinical trials.** *Am J Cardiol* 1988, **62**:1J–9J.
More recent appraisal of the same topic dealt with in [20].

22.   TYROLER HA: **Total serum cholesterol and ischemic heart disease risk in clinical trials and observational studies.** *Am J Prevent Med* 1985, **1**:18–24.

14

Epidemiological analysis of the prevention trials carried out before 1985.

23.   SCHUCKER B, WITTES JT, CUTLER JA, BAILEY K, MACKINTOSH DR, GORDON DJ, HAINES
       CM, MATTSON ME, GOOR RS, RIFKIND BM: **Change in physician perspective on
       cholesterol and heart disease. Results from two national surveys.** *JAMA* 1987,
       258:3521–3526.
Surveys of changes in US physicians' attitudes to the relevance of cholesterol-reduction in
preventing CHD.

24.   SCHUCKER B, BAILEY K, HEIMBACH JT, MATTSON ME, WITTES JT, HAINES CM, GORDON
       DJ, CUTLER JA, KEATING VS, GOOR RS, RIFKIND BM: **Change in public perspective
       on cholesterol and heart disease. Results from two national surveys.** *JAMA* 1987,
       258:3527–3531.
Analogous survey to that in [23] but involving members of the American public.

25.   KANNEL WB: **Contributions of the Framingham Study to the conquest of coronary
       artery disease.** *Am J Cardiol* 1988, **62**:1109–1112.
Summary of the impressive achievements made by the Framingham Study leading to a better
understanding of the aetiology of CHD and its prevention.

14

Index

Note: The following abbreviations have been used in the subentries of this index:
CHD, coronary heart disease; FCH, familial combined hyperlipidaemia; FH, familial
hypercholesterolaemia; HDL, high-density lipoprotein; LCAT, lecithin : cholesterol
acyltransferase; VLDL, very-low-density lipoprotein